Clinical Effectiveness in Nursing Practice

JANE DAWSON, RGN, RHV, MSC, PhD

Deputy Director, South West Cancer Intelligence Unit

with contributions from

ELAINE TAYLOR-WHILDE, MCSP, MIHSM, MA

Managing Director, ETW Research Consultants Ltd

SUE TORKINGTON, RGN, FWT, DIP N, PGCE, RNT

Head of Applied Social Sciences, Florence Nightingale School of
Nursing and Midwifery, King's College, London

LEEDS BECKETT UNIVERSITY
LIBRARY
DISCARDED

D0234159

W

WHURR PUBLISHERS

LONDON AND PHILADELPHIA

© 2001 Whurr Publishers
First published 2001 by
Whurr Publishers Ltd
19b Compton Terrace, London N1 2UN, England and
325 Chestnut Street, Philadelphia PA 19106, USA

Reprinted 2001

British Library Cataloguing in Publication Data
A catalogue record for this book is available from the
British Library.

ISBN: 1 86156 183 0

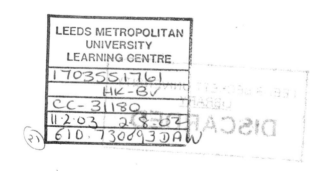
Printed and bound in the UK by Athenaeum Press Ltd,
Gateshead, Tyne & Wear

Contents

Introduction

Have you ever noticed how often a radio or television programme has an aspect of health care as its main subject, or includes a health-related item? Every television and radio channel is likely to include two or three health programmes a week and there will probably be at least one health item in programmes with a magazine format. Then there is the press. Women's magazines regularly run features and advice columns on health. Daily papers, both broadsheet and tabloid, also frequently have advice columns or a health journalist writing on matters of interest. Presumably, journalists and broadcasters pay so much attention to health care because they know – or assume – that the public are very interested.

When the NHS was introduced 50 years ago, the public's main concern was that healthcare would in the future be free to all, not just the prerogative of the rich. You could go to your doctor, tell him what was wrong and take the pills or medicine he (only very occasionally she) prescribed for you. The idea that you should ask your doctor what was the cause of your illness, how you could avoid it in future, what were the side effects of the medication and whether there was an alternative form of treatment just did not enter into it.

Today, all that has changed. Litigation for claims of negligence cost the NHS more each year. Complaints to the NHS Commissioner for Complaints are increasing and many more are resolved at hospital, primary care or health authority level. Patient groups exist in many general practices and there are numerous patient-related associations. Patients and the public now expect, indeed demand, to be involved in decisions, not just about their own health, but also in those affecting the community in which they live. In part, this has come about because people are better educated and more aware. It is also because, in the 50 years since it began, the NHS has become part of the nation's consciousness, an inherent cultural tradition. They 'pay' for it through taxes and National Insurance contributions, and the basic principles of fairness, equality of treatment and access to the best treatment regardless of cost, which underpinned the original legislation, are ones that the public treasure and expect to see fulfilled. So, when wards or hospitals close, community nurses reduce the hours of care they give and after-care facilities for the mentally ill are poor or non-existent, the public feel let down and want to know why this is happening. The current state of health services was one of the key issues in the 1997 General Election, which brought about a change of government after 18 years.

The reasons for this change of climate are complex. This book aims to examine some of them and to show how the emphasis on clinical effectiveness, evidence-based practice and clinical governance is all part of the changes in NHS policy, designed to make it more relevant and responsive to modern society. Chapter 1 sets the scene, considers what the term 'clinical effectiveness' means and examines how it fits into the context of clinical governance, whereas Chapter 2 explores the background and policy aspects related to improving health-care quality in more detail. Chapter 3 provides practical information on how to evaluate individual published research (reports, papers, etc.) as well as systematic reviews. Chapter 4 looks at the implications for nurse education and continuous professional development, and how these can be integrated into services. Chapter 5 considers the implications for nursing, particularly nurses' role and relationships with patients, other disciplines and the need for multidisciplinary working. Chapter 6 sets out some resources and ways of tapping into information.

There are some suggestions or 'challenges' for assignments that readers might like to try out for themselves as they read the book, to test out their understanding of the ideas examined. We hope the book will help nurses and other health-care workers to see how their clinical practice relates to the themes presented here.

Jane Dawson, Elaine Taylor-Whilde and Sue Torkington

Chapter 1
Background – how it all began

JANE DAWSON

The pace of technological and scientific discovery in health care is rapid, but new drugs and treatments are costly. People are living much longer – 70 is no longer considered particularly old, but as age increases so does the need for health care. The public hear of new medical discoveries and expect to receive them, driving up demands for services. The NHS is founded on the principle of equality of health care being available to all, but levels of service provision across the country are not equally distributed. No government, of whatever political persuasion, could hope to provide the resources needed for these developments without large increases in taxation, something that the public are not likely to welcome. The alternative strategy has been to examine closely the way that the NHS is run, with a view to targeting resources more effectively, reducing waste and controlling costs, the concept of 'value for money'. Although this has become a consistent theme in recent years, there have been two different but overlapping approaches to achieving this goal. The first has become known as 'corporate governance', and the second 'clinical governance'. To understand the meaning and context of clinical effectiveness, we need to look back and see how these two approaches run through NHS policy since the early 1980s.

Corporate governance

The idea of corporate governance is not confined to the NHS but can be applied to any business, or indeed social, institution. It simply means that those running such institutions have to provide good management and sound financial control of the enterprise. Although

1

the term 'corporate governance' was not used explicitly until later on, many policy decisions in the 1980s and 1990s can be seen as the start of efforts to introduce the concept to the NHS.

During its long term in office, the Conservative Government focused attention on management of the NHS. Clearly, sound management and financial control (corporate governance) are unlikely if the management systems in place are poor or inade-quately executed. After a review of the NHS, the Government published a White Paper in January 1989 (Department of Health, 1989) and passed the NHS Act 1990 (Clinical Outcomes Group, 1990). This was designed to improve efficiency and quality of care through the introduction of business principles and concepts, includ-ing the idea of a 'managed market' of purchasers and providers, to what was in effect a nationalised industry. Although this approach undoubtedly made great improvements to the overall efficiency of the NHS, it was not popular with clinicians, including nurses (Department of Health and Social Security, 1984). The United Kingdom Central Council for Nursing, Midwifery and Health Visit-ing (UKCC) drew up a supplement on professional accountability (UKCC, 1989) to the Code of Professional Practice (UKCC, 1992). This made it clear that professionals retained a duty of accountabil-ity for clinical practice and must 'seek to achieve and maintain high standards'. Managerial reorganisation did not, however, directly address the issue of the quality of clinical care that patients actually received. So it could be argued that the NHS became much more efficient at providing health care without knowing the extent to which the care given made any difference to health status.

In part, this had come about precisely because previous clinical autonomy gave clinicians the right to deliver the type of treatment they wanted to, in the manner they thought best, with no challenge to the how and why of that decision, in a public service that had to be accountable for its use of public resources. Day and Klein (1987) defined this dichotomy as attempting to 'combine the doctrine of public accountability with the doctrine of professional autonomy'. The White Paper of 1989 (Department of Health, 1989) had pointed out that there were wide variations between different parts of the NHS. For example, average costs of acute hospital stay could vary by 50%, even allowing for differences in types of patients being treated. Waiting times for operations and referral rates and prescribing by GPs were also given as examples of variation in performance. One of the key measures introduced by the 1990 NHS Act, which was aimed at tackling these issues, was that of medical audit. Chapter 2 considers medical audit in the context of other quality improvement programmes, but it is worth considering here how and why it came about.

Medical and clinical audit

The White Paper states the intention of medical audit:

> To ensure that all who deliver patient services make the best use of resources, quality of service and value for money will be more rigorously audited. Arrangements for medical audit by peer review will be extended throughout the NHS.
>
> Department of Health (January 1989)

The White Paper was followed by a series of 'Working Papers'. Working Paper 6 set out the arrangements to establish medical audit and a sum of £250 000 was made available in 1989–90 (Secretaries of State for Social Services, 1989). Crucially, although Working Paper 6 stated that medical audit should be clinically led, it also made clear that:

> Every doctor should participate in regular systematic medical audit.

Although medical audit was to be essentially a professional matter, managers, who had a responsibility for the effective use of resources, would need to ensure that effective medical audit was in place in their hospital or community trust. Systems were also established to encourage audit within primary care. Whether or not individual practitioners examined the quality of their care was no longer purely a professional decision, but a matter for legitimate managerial concern and interest. In other words, a managerial process was introduced with the expectation that it would improve the efficiency and effectiveness of health care. The principle of corporate governance is discernible here in the duty, which was firmly laid on managers and trust boards, to ensure proper arrangements to support a clinical matter.

Professional organisations could not ignore such developments and increasingly became proactive in the field of audit. Indeed, some professional organisations had already recognised that this was an integral part of their role and had instigated, supported and encouraged initiatives such as quality programmes, and national and local audit, as well as providing education on the new techniques required by audit. The Royal College of Physicians (1989) supported the widespread development of medical audit, the Royal College of Surgeons undertook the Confidential Enquiry into Perioperative Deaths (Buck, Devlin and Lunn, 1987) and the Royal College of Radiologists (1988) had conducted studies into the appropriate use of radiological investigations. In 1990, the Royal College of Nursing began a major initiative to educate and support nurses in the development of standards of care (Royal College of Nursing, 1989).

As medical audit was gradually set in motion, it became clear that audit of clinical care had to involve other health-care professionals, not just doctors. Funding became available specifically for clinical audit from 1992, although in many areas medical audit had already begun to involve other disciplines.

So what is medical/clinical audit and did it achieve what it was intended to achieve? Working Paper 6 (Secretaries of State for Social Services, 1989) defines medical audit as:

> The systematic, critical analysis of the quality of medical care, including the procedures used for diagnosis and treatment, the use of resources and the resulting outcome and quality of life for the patient.

This definition was not appropriate once other health-care disciplines became involved in the audit process, nor did it take into account patients' perspectives. A number of definitions were used, but the most generally acceptable is that by Moss (1992):

> the systematic critical analysis of the quality of clinical care, by all those who contribute to care. It includes the procedures used for diagnosis and treatment, the use of resources and the resulting quality of life for the patient – for this the patient's views must be sought. Its objectives are improvements in the quality of clinical practice.

The NHS Executive (Department of Health, 1989) set out the fundamental principles of clinical audit in the box.

Clinical audit

- Clinical audit is professionally led and essentially an educational process
- It should become an inevitable part of routine clinical practice
- It uses standard setting as a basis for audit activity
- It has a patient focus and a patient/carer input
- It is undertaken by clinical teams
- It involves general management to help ensure that health gains inform audit activity
- It must retain confidentiality at the patient and clinician level
- It will inform purchasing strategies
- It is linked to the 'Health of the Nation' agenda, strategic issues and needs assessment

---

Examination of these principles reveals fairly quickly that they are contradictory. How could clinical audit retain confidentiality if general managers were to use it to ensure health gain? If it was to inform purchasing strategies, how could it be essentially an educational process? Initially, funds for supporting medical, then clinical, audit had been channelled through Regional Health Authorities so that audit developed and operated in a protected environment. In 1994–95, this changed and resources were passed over to District Health Authorities and Family Health Services Authorities (purchasers), which began to develop contracts for clinical audit with the NHS trusts and GPs (providers) in their area.

The dichotomies in the purpose of clinical audit mentioned above became heightened. Health-care professionals began to question the purpose of the huge amount of time and effort required to maintain an effective clinical audit programme, and managers considered that clinical audit had been less effective in bringing about changes in services than had been hoped (Maynard, 1991). Alongside this, there were a number of separate but interrelated policy developments, which shifted the focus from looking simply at *what* was done towards looking at the research evidence on which health care was based.

In part, clinicians have always examined research findings to guide them in practice. This is particularly the case in medicine, where clinical trials of new drugs and treatments are an everyday event, although other health professionals such as nurses and therapists have increasingly been drawn into research to guide and inform practice. However, implementation of research into clinical practice has always been a major problem (Humphris and Littlejohns, 1996) and this is particularly so in nursing (Closs and Cheater, 1994; Dunn et al., 1994; English, 1994; Walsh, 1997). Clinical audit itself began to bring about a change in this, because audit of clinical performance in relation to what *had* been done could be conducted only in comparison with what *ought* to be done. Thus, clinical audit staff and health-care professionals found themselves increasingly drawn in to the process of searching the research literature for evidence from which to set standards for audit. In 1989, the Royal College of Nursing (RCN, 1989) defined standards as the following:

Professionally agreed levels of performance for a particular population which is

- Achievable
- Observable
- Desirable
- Measurable.

The RCN went on to describe the sources for developing standards as:

- professional experience
- values and beliefs
- legal requirements
- policies, procedures and guidelines for practice
- management: mission statements, learning objectives
- published research findings.

The development of standards takes a great deal of time. In addition, research evidence does not always exist or may be contradictory, so professional experience and consensus can play a more prominent role. This is then a question of personal opinion and values. What if members of a clinical team disagree as to how best to treat a particular condition or group of patients?

The role and use of research

One of the most important developments was a change in the way research in health care was coordinated and funded. Previously, money for conducting research was available from a wide variety of sources: the Medical Research Council, Regional Health Authorities, charitable funds, Royal Colleges, etc. All these bodies worked independently and could very well be funding similar research. In 1993, the Government set out a Research and Development Strategy (Department of Health, 1993) with the aim of coordinating the resources available and avoiding duplication of effort. Furthermore, it was intended that, in future, research would be directed at answering or examining questions that had a major bearing on the health of the population or particular sectors of the population. As a result of this, scientific evidence about health care began to focus more on questions of the clinical effectiveness and cost-effectiveness of clinical practice. The interrelationship of research, policy and clinical care is discussed further in Chapter 2.

Another factor was the increasing recognition that evidence for or against a particular drug or treatment was not always black and white. Frequently, research findings differed or were inconclusive. A method of overcoming this, known as systematic review, became increasingly prominent and a number of academic centres (York and Oxford) began to develop expertise in this field and to teach the skills to others (Sheldon and Chalmers, 1994). We return to this in Chapter 3.

In 1993, the NHS Executive set up the NHS Health Technology Assessment (HTA) programme (NHS Executive, 1998). Its purpose was to examine the effectiveness of new interventions in the NHS in the light of research evidence, whereas previously new health technologies had all too frequently been introduced before there was comprehensive and reliable information or assessment of their clinical and cost-effectiveness.

A further strand was the setting up of the Clinical Standards Advisory Group (NHS and Community Care Act 1990) to act as an independent source of advice to health ministers and the NHS generally on standards of care. This multidisciplinary group focuses on a particular condition (cystic fibrosis, community health care for elderly people) and examines how services are provided by different health authorities and trusts. It then makes recommendations on how service outcomes can be improved – in other words, how to make them more clinically effective, by developing what are known as clinical guidelines. These are discussed in more detail later in the chapter

The evolution of the clinical effectiveness agenda

The emphasis and drive to ensure that care is clinically effective have not been a sudden, overnight shift, but a gradual evolution over a period of time and through a variety of policies and organisational mechanisms. The NHS Strategy White Paper *A Service with Ambitions* (Secretary of State for Health, 1996) set out the key principles of equity, effectiveness and responsiveness, and was followed by a series of NHS E publications including an Executive Letter (NHS E, 1995) 'Improving the effectiveness of clinical services'. The letter stated that [EL (95) 105]:

> Improving the clinical effectiveness of NHS services is one of the most important ways in which we can secure significant improvements to the health of the people of England.

It summarised how sources of information, clinical guidelines, clinical audit and HTA all contributed to improving clinically effective health care. The document that accompanied the EL, *Promoting Clinical Effectiveness. A Framework for Action in and through the NHS* (NHS E, 1996b), set out the role of health authorities, NHS trusts and clinicians, and established a framework of inform, monitor, change. This sought to bring together, in a cohesive form, the various initiatives already taking place which all had the goal of improving the effectiveness of clinical care.

The framework for clinical effectiveness

Just what did this framework mean and what is clinical effectiveness? The framework defines clinical effectiveness as [EL (95) 105]:

> The extent to which specific clinical interventions, when deployed in the field for a particular patient or population, do what they are intended to do – ie maintain and improve health and secure the greatest possible gain from available resources. (NHS E, 1995)

Let us look at how that might apply in practice. If a doctor gives a patient a particular drug, does it either resolve the condition, or at least keep it stable? Antibiotics are given to combat specific infections and the expectation is that the infection will be overcome and the patient gets better. Patients with diabetes require insulin and/or dietary regimens, not because the diabetes will go away, but to keep it stable. Research and experience have shown these treatments to be clinically effective. Increasingly, nurses are also being challenged to demonstrate that nursing interventions are based on evidence of effectiveness. Some years ago, one routine preventive measure for pressure sores was to massage the areas at risk (heels, elbows and buttocks) with methylated spirit and talcum powder! Research showed that this was not effective (Young and Dobranski, 1992); indeed, it was detrimental to skin integrity, so this procedure has been stopped. What was shown to be effective was accurate assessment of risk, good nutrition, and pressure-relieving devices and frequent changes of position (Breslaw, 1991). Similarly, there were many strange nursing practices in relation to leg ulcers, from the application of various potions (honey, egg-white) to exposing the ulcer to a hair dryer. Again, research demonstrated that such practices did not improve the condition (Moffat and Dorman, 1994) and they have now (hopefully) been discontinued or not continued because it has become an accepted routine – 'We've always done it like that' or 'Sister likes it done'.

This brings us to another dimension to effectiveness, namely cost-effectiveness. The NHS E document *Promoting Clinical Effectiveness* (NHS E, 1996b) says that:

> The cost effectiveness of a particular form of health care depends upon the ratio of the costs of health care to its health outcomes. Cost effectiveness is central to the meaning of 'clinical effectiveness' in this booklet, except where a more specific reference is made at appropriate points in the text. Only by choosing more cost effective services are we able to secure the greatest possible health gain from the resources available.

> **Challenge**: Can you think of examples in your everyday practice where there is little or no evidence that the treatment will make any difference at all to the patient's health status? Ask your colleagues their opinion as to why these are still carried out.

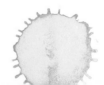

In other words, it is not just a question of what does and what does not work, but how costly it is in relation to the improvement in health. If a patient's condition could be improved in 2 weeks by a particular treatment that was extremely expensive, but would get better in 2.5 weeks even if untreated, then use of the treatment is not cost-effective. Not providing adequate pressure-relieving mattresses in an orthopaedic ward may be cheaper in the short term but, if the number of bed-days taken through pressure sores increases substantially, it is not a cost-effective form of care. If two treatments have similar outcomes, but one is half the cost of the other, the cheaper of the two is the most clinically (and cost) effective.

The same rationale must be applied to interventions aimed at populations. Immunisation and vaccination programmes are clinically effective and cost-effective, because the consequences of treating the illnesses that would arise if such programmes were discontinued outweigh the cost of implementing them, to say nothing of the human suffering and distress. It is now possible to screen populations for the presence of a number of conditions but, if the chances of having the disease are very small, or there is no effective treatment anyway, such screening would not be clinically effective or cost-effective. So the drive to ensure the clinical effectiveness of care is the next and logical development in a series of attempts to provide better health care to all those who need it, within the resources available, by eliminating ineffective interventions and encouraging the application of interventions known to be clinically effective. It is in fact an element of corporate governance, i.e. the duty to manage health care and its costs efficiently and prudently.

The three stages – inform, change and monitor – set out in the framework document (NHS E, 1996b) are interdependent in the process of implementing a cohesive approach to more clinically effective health care. We consider each in turn to see what they mean in – and for – practice.

Inform

Unless clinicians have good evidence about what is the best way to treat patients or organise services, they cannot attempt to make them more clinically effective. This evidence will come from research, but also from information about how many people need a service, what resources are available and how care is currently delivered. A key issue here is that the information must be readily accessible and up to date. Busy doctors and nurses simply do not have the time to spend searching the literature to try to identify evidence for clinical practice. Librarians are, however, increasingly providing searching and synthesising services, current awareness lists and other facilities. Bodies such as the Royal College of Nursing are involved in the development and collation of guidelines and other information, based on evidence of best practice. Professional journals are another source of information and a number of journals, e.g. *British Journal for Clinical Governance*, have been set up in recent years as a source of information and education. Chapter 6 deals in detail with the question of how to find the information you need and the various initiatives designed to make the process easier.

Challenge: Choose a condition or practice situation relevant to your clinical area. What facilities does your trust or clinical service have to allow you to look at how best to treat your patients? Do you have access to a library? Is there a link to the Internet, NHSnet or other computer facilities? Does the library or anywhere else in your organisation keep a list of relevant publications to enable you to keep up to date?

Change

Once clinicians have accessed the available information and made decisions about how their practice or service could become more clinically effective, a programme for change must be put in place. Certain factors must be present, however, if the change is to be implemented successfully. Simply deciding that 'things will be different' just will not do!

- Change must be instigated and managed at a local level. Only those practitioners and managers involved with the particular service or clinical area can bring about meaningful change. Imposition may work for a time, but is unlikely to be sustained if those 'on the ground' are not truly supportive.
- Change needs the agreement and cooperation of all within the clinical team. It is no good one member of a department deciding to change practice if colleagues are unaware of or even disagree

with the change. Consensus must be reached, so that all members of the team understand what is required of them and how their practice fits in.

• Change must be planned. How and in what way clinical practice or service delivery are to be changed must be thought through carefully. Is there a timetable of planned events? Who is responsible for what? What are the consequences for the clinical team, for other colleagues, for other departments or services? Have they been informed? Have patients been informed? It is here that the use of clinical guidelines can be helpful. There are a number of different definitions of guidelines. The NHS E, in its publication *Clinical Guidelines. Using Clinical Guidelines to Improve Patient Care within the NHS* (NHS E, 1996a) states that they are:

Systematically developed statements which assist clinicians and patients in making decisions about appropriate treatment for specific conditions.

Another definition (Institute for Medicine, 1992) is:

Systematically developed statements to assist practitioner and client decisions about appropriate health care for specific clinical circumstances.

You'll notice that both these definitions use the word 'systematically'. This brings us back to the earlier discussion about the nature of research evidence. As well as being systematic, guidelines should have the other characteristics in the box.

All this sounds very complicated but the NHS E publication (NHS E, 1996a) states that: 'Clinical guidelines are produced for one reason and one reason only: to improve the quality of care.' If you look through the list you will see that all those features need to be present if guidelines are to support evidence-based practice, which has exactly that aim.

How are guidelines developed?

Guidelines can be developed at a national or a local level.

National

We have already considered one route by which guidelines are developed, namely through work such as that by the Clinical Outcomes Group. As well as this body, professional organisations may produce and distribute guidelines to their members. There are

---

Characteristics of guidelines

Validity: Use of the guidelines should lead to the expected results. The outcomes for patients of applying the guidelines should be what clinicians hoped to achieve.

Reproducibility: Would another group of clinicians develop the same guidelines, given that they used the same evidence? In other words, the guidelines are not based on personal opinion, prejudice or some 'hidden agenda'.

Reliability: Will different professionals interpret and implement the guidelines in the same way, given the same clinical circumstances? If guidelines are open to misinterpretation, then neither clinicians nor patients can really know what to expect.

Representative: Those with a central interest in the topic must have been involved in development of the guidelines.

Clinically applicable: It is clear to which group of patients the guidelines refer.

Flexibility: Not all patients are exactly the same even when they have the same clinical diagnosis. Guidelines should take this into account and identify exceptions.

Clarity: It should be easy for clinicians and patients to understand what the guidelines say. Unnecessary use of jargon and technical terms should be avoided.

Reviewable: Research evidence, patients' expectations, organisations and circumstances change over time. Guidelines need to be reviewed regularly to see that they are still relevant.

Capable of audit: It should be possible to develop criteria by which the use of the guidelines can be audited.

---

a number of centres, such as the NHS Centre for Reviews and Dissemination based at the University of York and the Cochrane Centre, which carry out the systematic review of literature on which the guidelines can be based. Chapter 3 looks at systematic reviews in more detail and explains how they are conducted and how they can be appraised.

Local

Sometimes, guidelines produced at the national level can be adopted as they stand for local implementation, although almost invariably some adaptations will be required to reflect local circumstances, needs and opinions. In addition, if one professional group has developed the guidelines, multidisciplinary discussion will be needed to see how their use will affect the clinical team as a whole, and then the guidelines need to be extended to take this into account. Alternatively, local clinicians may decide to develop their own guidelines. But beware! The process takes a great deal of time and effort and requires people with the necessary skills. It is always advisable to make use of existing material if at all possible.

Challenge: Can you find a clinical guideline for use in your speciality? How was it developed? Is it already in use? If not, what would be needed to bring about its implementation? What other groups – clinicians, patients, other agencies – would need to be involved?

Arguably, giving care to a patient without being aware of the possible outcome could be said to be unethical.

Monitor

It would obviously be pointless to go to great effort to find evidence of best practice, put into effect the changes required, and then just hope for the best. So there have to be systems of monitoring in place to see what the effect of all this is. Change is rarely smooth and there may well be difficulties in implementation, which are unlikely to be addressed unless the results are measured carefully. In addition, you need to find out just what the outcome has been for patients.

Monitoring can be done at a number of different levels. Let us take an example of a clinic for people with diabetes. Evidence suggests that patients with diabetes are most receptive to advice on diet when they are newly diagnosed, rather than when they run into difficulty (Cradock, 1996). They are more likely to follow the advice and achieve better diabetic control, lessening the risk of both short- and long-term complications. The staff at a health centre decide that, in future, all patients with diabetes attending the clinic will be seen by the dietitian attached to the centre. Six months later, the clinical team plan to monitor what is happening. How could they do this? For a start, the question could be asked: 'Have the planned changes actually taken place?' A patient survey or analysis of the dietitian's clinic returns will easily provide the answer. If it is not happening, why not? Perhaps the clinic time is too short, or maybe there is no relief cover when the dietitian is sick or on leave.

At the next level, the question could be: 'Are patients following the advice given and is their diabetic control better?' Again, a patient survey would probably answer the first part, but more careful investigation would be required for the second. You might see how often newly diagnosed patients had visited their GP since diagnosis, assuming that if all were well they would not need to keep returning. You could find out whether any of them had attended the local accident and emergency department for diabetes-related problems, or whether any had experienced a hypoglycaemic coma. These can be seen as 'proxy' measures, but a more direct measure would be to look regularly at glucose blood levels over a period of time to see whether they were stable and within normal limits.

Finally, what have been the longer-term benefits of this new practice? It could be extrapolated that, if patients with diabetes maintain optimum control over a period of years, they should suffer fewer complications, such as hypoglycaemic comas, and even life-threatening events such as leg ulceration or amputation, and require lower levels of medication. Clearly this would require follow-up over a much longer time period and, in any case, other variables will come into play.

The point to remember is that, as well as monitoring the practical aspects of change, i.e. did it happen as planned, the objective of monitoring is to demonstrate the following:

- Health has been improved
- The improvement is the result of the intervention.

This is a very simple example. Fairly straightforward methods of measurement, such as patient surveys, clinical audit and drug monitoring, could be employed to gauge the effectiveness of such an intervention. You can see, however, that in some cases monitoring for the health benefit of a treatment claimed to be more clinically effective requires very sophisticated measurement. For a start, what aspect of health would you measure – improvement in clinical signs and symptoms, increased mobility and function or death? Is the benefit greater than would have been achieved by other, perhaps cheaper or simpler, treatment? Another problem is that, up till now, the NHS has not been good at routinely collecting or linking the kind of information needed to answer these questions, especially over a longer time frame. More recently, the development of information strategies and increasing computerisation are beginning to address this issue.

Challenge: Consider the guideline you found for your clinical area. What measures can you think of which could be used to monitor its implementation and outcomes?

You can see that although the inform, change, monitor framework is a relatively straightforward concept, putting it into practice at all levels of the NHS is an extremely complex and demanding task. Although such things as improved information systems, guidelines, research and literature reviews all have a vital part to play, the most significant development has been the introduction of clinical governance.

Clinical governance

In some ways, making a clear distinction between corporate and clinical governance is misleading, or at least conveys a less than accurate picture. You can probably see that the execution of corporate governance initially placed the emphasis on having systems in place in which clinical staff were expected to operate in order to improve management of resources and quality of care. The objective of all the policies described above, such as clinical audit, a focused research and development strategy, systematic reviews, development of guidelines, etc. was to improve the quality of health care. However, by increment, they began to introduce the concept of clinical governance, albeit implicitly.

In May 1997, a Labour Government was elected to office and one of its first actions was to publish a White Paper (Department of Health, 1997) on the new NHS. Although this set out a new management structure for health care and abolished the managed market principle, one of its major changes was to make health-care organisations accountable not just for good management and financial control, but also for the standard of clinical care itself – something that until then had been seen as primarily a professional matter. Clinical governance thus became an explicit and statutory responsibility of trusts, health authorities and the newly introduced primary care groups, for which they would in future be accountable.

Clinical governance is a new term to many and, as such, the implications are very much under examination and are still the subject of attempts to arrive at a clear and comprehensive definition. The White Paper (Department of Health, 1997) stated that clinical governance is:

> A new initiative . . . to assure and improve clinical standards at local level throughout the NHS. This includes action to ensure that risks are avoided, adverse events are rapidly detected . . . good practice is rapidly disseminated and systems are in place to ensure continuous improvements in clinical care.

Donaldson (1998) suggests that clinical governance is:

> A framework through which NHS organisations are accountable for continuously improving the quality of their services and safeguarding their high standards of care by creating an environment in which clinical excellence in clinical care will flourish

whereas Dunning and Ayres (1998) consider that:

> Clinical Governance places expectations and responsibilities on individuals and organisations to put in place systems to ensure the delivery of high quality health care to patients.

This is a debate that has just started and that will progress alongside ideas and initiatives for implementation. Clinical governance is not one specific event or item. It is in fact a 'catch-all' phrase that covers a whole range of issues, a kind of framework to improve care in the NHS. Thus, it both builds on and strengthens the concepts introduced in the *Promoting Clinical Effectiveness* document (NHS E, 1996b).

Dale et al. (1998) argue that the 'Four Pillars' of clinical governance are: improving clinical effectiveness, professional development, continuous quality improvement and risk management. We have already begun to consider the issues surrounding clinical effectiveness, what that involves and how this is aimed at ensuring that the clinical practice of all health professionals is evidence-based. Let us now turn to the other three of Dale's 'Pillars'.

Risk management

Risk management will be considered in more detail in a later chapter but, in brief, the term covers a range of activities and policies that are designed to encourage good practice and prevent things going wrong. This should include the anticipation and prevention of potential problems, such as extra demands on beds or services, staff shortages, equipment breakdowns, etc. Good risk management will use critical incidents (patient accidents, drug or treatment errors) and patient complaints in a positive manner, not just as a reason to 'blame' staff, as well as to empower clinical staff to develop their practice. This leads us on to the other two 'Pillars': professional development and continuous quality improvement.

Professional development

Staff cannot deliver good care if they do not have the necessary skills and competence to do so. That means that there must be opportunities for training, not just at the basic level necessary for qualification, but throughout their careers, so that staff can update their knowledge and refresh their thinking. Poor performance should be recognised and staff helped to learn from their mistakes. All too often the NHS operates a culture of blame and negative criticism and this must be turned around. There are implications for workload here, because clinical services are delivered over 24 hours, all year round, and in future this cannot be a justification for denying clinical staff the opportunity to attend training courses or take study days. The issue of arrangements to support clinical supervision and the development of clinical leadership skills come in here as well.

Continuous quality improvement

Most NHS trusts, community services and GP practices will already have some arrangements in place, such as a committee or team with responsibility for 'quality'. Unfortunately, this can mean anything and everything. In the context of clinical governance, it should mean having appropriate mechanisms in place for the constant examination of and working towards improvement in the quality of care and the way in which it is delivered throughout the organisation. There are no 'quick fixes' here. It requires a culture of openness and trust, in which staff can openly discuss their practice, reflect upon what is good and not so good, and draw up plans for improvement.

These 'Four Pillars' are considered in more detail in later chapters, but you can probably see from all this that many of the required systems for clinical governance already exist within health service organisations. Clinical governance simply pulls them all together, collating reports on quality issues, training needs, risk management, etc. to arrive at an overall picture on standards of clinical care. How this is to be done in practice will differ between organisations and depend on the arrangements and structures already in place. What suits a primary care group may not be applicable to an acute NHS trust, or to a mental health service. However, clinical governance should not automatically lead to the establishment of a new 'Clinical Governance Committee'.

Clinical governance and the delivery of care that is clinically effective will require a change in attitude, both for clinicians of all disciplines and for managers. However, if managers are to be accountable for the standard of clinical care in their organisation, then doctors, nurses, midwives and therapists must be accountable for the clinical effectiveness of their practice. Dialogue will be essential – clinicians must be prepared to set priorities, examine current practice critically and be explicit about what changes are required, the resources needed to bring that about and the expected benefits for patients. Managers must be able to understand the concerns of clinicians and patients, ensure organisational systems and resources, support clinical governance and join in constructive debate about how to achieve improvements.

Challenge: Find out what structures and committees already exist within your trust, clinical service or GP practice that have a remit of audit, quality, risk management, complaints or some other aspect of examining standards of care. Think how these could be brought together or coordinated to implement clinical governance, then find out what is actually happening to bring this about.

Across the board there are a number of initiatives proposed or already in place:

- NHS trusts and GPs are increasingly working with health authorities to define the most clinically effective practice for specified conditions, e.g. diabetes and asthma, then collecting data systematically to measure outcome.
- Data sets are available at a national level to allow comparison between different population groups.
- A 'Health Outcome Indicators Programme' has been set up to develop indicators for a number of topics.
- A National Institute for Clinical Excellence was introduced in the 1997 NHS White Paper, number 32, (DoH 1997).
- Outcome scales have been described for the 'Health of the Nation' targets.
- National audits are being encouraged and set up.
- Different ways of grouping patients with similar health problems are being explored.
- The Clinical Standards Advisory Group has a programme to look at standards and practice in various NHS trusts and other settings, and has published a number of reports.

It is too soon to say just how health authorities, NHS trusts and primary care groups, introduced by the White Paper (DoH 1997), will respond in order to meet their new roles and responsibilities, but it is clear that major changes in both organisational structures and culture are in progress. What is also generally accepted (Kitson, 1998; Wilcock, 1998), as central to the concept of clinical governance is the importance of teams and teamwork. This will not apply just to clinical teams working within their own specific departments and specialties, but must become multidisciplinary, extend outside the clinical environment to other clinical settings (primary/secondary) to managerial systems and departments (planning, personnel) and even to other agencies (social services, housing).

There is a lot happening in the field of health policy and development, all aimed at improving the quality of health care through the delivery of care that is cost-effective and clinically effective, but it is a vast and never-ending task and many of the policies and initiatives will take years to work through to health care at the everyday level.

However, there is no viable alternative. The status quo is simply no longer an option.

The changing role of patients

We started this chapter by considering how patient and public expectations have changed since the inception of the NHS 50 years ago. What we have not discussed is the way that recognition of this and of the increased involvement of patients (and carers) in decisions concerning healthcare are woven through many of the policy changes of the last 20 years. The idea of a partnership between patients, the public and those working in the NHS in decision-making has been introduced and will in future be central in consideration of how clinical care is to be delivered in future. Clinical governance is part of that change because it must affect patients and the wider public. Standards of care will be more clearly stated and mechanisms for gaining patients' opinions are now integrated into organisational systems and given serious thought. In Chapter 5, we look in more detail at health policy from this angle and consider the involvement of patients within the context of partnerships with multiagency and multidisciplinary teams.

Conclusions

In this chapter, we have seen that the drive to improve clinical effectiveness is not just one 'magic bullet' approach to better quality of health care. It has come about almost sequentially over a period of several years, and will no doubt take many more years before it is embedded as a basic principle of clinical practice. The clinical effectiveness policy at the national level covers a wide range of mechanisms, strategies and programmes. However, the NHS is made up of individual health-care professionals, so each one has a part to play. The thing to remember is that, even if you think you have no involvement in these national programmes and policy changes, you have a professional duty to reflect on the clinical effectiveness of your practice.

References

Breslaw R (1991) Nutritional status and dietary intake of patients with pressure ulcers: review of the research literature 1943 to 1989. Decubitus 1: 16–21.

Buck N, Devlin HB, Lunn JN (1987) Report of a Confidential Enquiry into Peri-operative Deaths. London: Nuffield Provincial Hospitals Trust and King's Fund.

Clinical Outcomes Group (1990) Section 62, National Health Service and Community Care Act 1990. London: HMSO.

Closs SJ, Cheater F (1994) Utilization of nursing research: culture, interest and support. Journal of Advanced Nursing 19: 762–73.

Cradock S (1996) Answers to nurses' questions on diet and diabetes. Community Nurse 2(8): 31–2.

Dale R, Croft A, Kenyon M (1998) Implementing clinical governance. Healthcare Quality 4(3): 22–5.

Day P, Klein R (1987) Accountabilities: Five Public Services. London: Tavistock Publications.

Department of Health (1989) White Paper 'Working for Patients'. Cd 555. London: HMSO.

Department of Health (1990) National Health Service and Community Care Act. London: HMSO.

Department of Health (1993) Research for Health. London: HMSO.

Department of Health (1997) NHS England: The New NHS – Modern and Dependable. London: NHS Executive.

Department of Health and Social Security (1984) The Next Steps: Management in the Health Service, para 6. London: DHSS.

Donaldson LJ (1998) Clinical governance: a statutory duty for quality improvement. Journal of Epidemiology Community Health 52: 73–4.

Dunn EV, Norton PG, Stewart M, Tudiver F, Bass MJ (1994) Disseminating Research/Changing practice. Thousand Oaks, CA: SAGE.

Dunning M, Ayres P (1998) What is clinical governance? – a workable definition. Healthcare Quality 4(3): 16–18.

English I (1994) Nursing as a research based profession: 22 years after Briggs. British Journal of Nursing 3: 402–6.

Humphris D, Littlejohns P (1996) Implementing clinical guidelines: preparation and opportunism. Journal of Clinical Effectiveness 1(1): 5–7.

Institute for Medicine (1992) Guidelines for Clinical Practice: From Development to Use. Washington, DC: National Academy Press.

Kitson A (1998) The Government White Papers: A view from nursing. Healthcare Quality 4(1): 5–9.

Maynard A (1991) The case for auditing audit. Health Services Journal 101(526): 26.

Moffat C, Dorman M (1994) Recurrence of leg ulcers within the community ulcer service. Journal of Wound Care 4(2): 57–61.

Moss F (1992) Achieving quality in hospital practice. Quality in Health Care Suppl (1) 17–19.

NHS E (1995) Improving the Effectiveness of Clinical Services. EL (95) 105. Leeds: Department of Health.

NHS E (1996a) Clinical Guidelines: Using Clinical Guidelines to Improve Patient Care within the NHS. London: Department of Health.

NHS E (1996b) Promoting Clinical Effectiveness. A Framework for Action in and through the NHS. London: HMSO.

NHS E (1998) The Annual Report of the NHS Health Technology Assessment Programme 1998. London: Department of Health.

Royal College of Nursing (1989) Standards of Care: A Framework for Quality. Harrow: Scutari.

Royal College of Physicians of London (1989) Medical Audit: a Final Report – What, Why and How. London: Royal College of Physicians of London.

Royal College of Radiologists (1988) Annotation: towards the more effective use of diagnostic radiology: a review of the work of the Royal College of Radiologists Working Party on the more effective use of diagnostic radiology 1976–1986. Clinical Radiology 39: 3–6.

Secretaries of State for Social Services (1989) Working for Patients. Working Paper 6. Cd 555. London: HMSO.

Secretary of State for Health (1996) The National Health Service: A Service with Ambitions. London: HMSO.

Sheldon T, Chalmers I (1994) The UK Cochrane Centre and the NHS Centre for reviews and dissemination: Respective roles within the information systems strategy of the NHS R&D programme, co-ordination and principles underlying collaboration. Health Economist 3(3): 201–3.

United Kingdom Central Council for Nursing, Midwifery and Health Visiting (1989) Exercising Accountability. London: UKCC.

United Kingdom Central Council for Nursing, Midwifery and Health Visiting (1992) Code of Professional Conduct. London: UKCC.

Walsh M (1997) How nurses perceive barriers to research implementation. Nursing Standard 11(29): 34–9.

Wilcock P (1998) The new NHS: an opportunity for modern, quality thinking about quality improvement healthcare. Quality 4(1): 21–6.

Young JB, Dobranski S (1992) Pressure sores: epidemiological and current management concepts. Drugs and Ageing 2: 42–57

Chapter 2
Health policy

ELAINE TAYLOR-WHILDE

Health policy is intended to be a guiding influence, there for those who are responsible for delivering health services. As a student or practising healthcare professional, however, it can seem remote and alien to the environment in which we operate. The purpose of this chapter is to demonstrate that without policy there would not be a health service and indeed it can form a useful part within all our working lives. To understand the role of health policy, we look at where it has come from and some of the developments in health policy over the past 10 years. The chapter examines the most recent NHS policy in the 1997 NHS White Paper *The New NHS* (Department of Health, 1997a) and the new concepts clinical governance and primary care groups contained within it. We then explore in some detail its influence on practice and concentrate on how policy may be implemented.

We also look at the ultimate aim of health policy – to improve the health of the nation – and explore the inequalities in health that still prevail today, some 16 years after the publication of the Black Report *Inequalities in Health* (Black et al., 1992). We consider the impact of such policy documents as the Green Paper *Our Healthier Nation* (Department of Health, 1997b) and how initiatives such as Health Improvement Programmes and Health Action Zones can help achieve the targets for improved health contained within it.

One of the main issues within health policy is proactively to enable the voice of the public, patient and carer to be heard (NHS Executive, 1998). We shall see whether indeed this has been done and what effect it has had thus far.

Where has it come from?

If you don't know where you are going you may end up somewhere else.
Peter Homa, Chief Executive, Leicester Royal Infirmary (Homa, 1994)

Health policy is the basis from which strategies for healthcare services are developed. From these strategies, business plans are drawn up by all NHS health authorities, NHS trusts and the new primary care groups. Business plans set out in detail how the intentions in the strategy set by health care are actually to be delivered. It may be useful therefore to think of health policy as the start of the healthcare process. Clearly, there are political considerations, because the process inevitably starts with the government in place in the country concerned. Health is an emotive subject and one that is of great relevance to all – professionals and members of the public. Thus, health policy is developed by what may seem to some a surprisingly cyclical process, which takes account of a broad range of perspectives.

We must also bear in mind the effects of globalisation. With the advent of electronic communication and faster travel, world economies and cultures are no longer as radically different as they once were. For healthcare, the result has been that health systems are becoming broadly similar from country to country. An example of this is accreditation – a tick box system used for checking the quality of healthcare services. Accreditation, once barely encountered outside the USA, is now widely seen throughout the westernised countries, including the UK. Worldwide influences affect UK health policy, in particular that flowing from organisations such as the World Health Organisation and World Bank. New political changes such as the development of the European Economic Union also affect the way in which the member states develop their healthcare systems. Much funding flows from the European Union and changes in working practice and European law all have an impact on UK health care.

In the UK, the body responsible for setting healthcare policy is the Department of Health. In England, the Permanent Secretary, accountable to the Secretary of State for Health (SoS), the lead Government minister, heads the Department of Health (DoH). The SoS has a team of Ministers who are advised by special advisers and civil servants. Now part of the DoH is the NHS Executive, the NHS headquarters headed by a Chief Executive, together with a senior team including the Chief Nursing and Medical Officers. These advisers draw considerable expertise from the health service itself and from academics and special advisory groups. Indeed, at any one time a number of civil servants within the NHS headquarters have NHS backgrounds, being either clinically or managerially qualified. In Scotland, Wales and Northern Ireland, there are separate but similar systems, each led by its own minister.

In areas where there is particular difficulty or concern, e.g. the National Centre for Clinical Excellence and Clinical Negligence, special health authorities have been set up to administer and run detailed systems. Again the teams running these health authorities are experts in the areas concerned. Both these health authorities were created with the main purpose of improving the quality of healthcare within the UK and are examined in detail later in the chapter

Much health policy is actually created by NHS staff. An example of this was EL (93) 110 *Achieving An Organisation Wide Approach to Quality* (NHS Executive, 1993) which originated from an example of best practice from Hertfordshire. Special teams of NHS experts (in this case the then Regional Quality lead) take these examples of best practice and advise civil servants how best to promulgate them throughout the health service.

Although creating health policy is difficult, achieving the successful implementation of it in the form of evidence-based guidelines is by far the most difficult task. Implementing evidence-based health care requires experienced change management skills and a concerted marketing effort, which traditionally the NHS lacks (Figure 2.1). This has already been touched on in Chapter 1.

Challenge: See if you can find out the distribution chain in your trust for information sent out from the Department of Health. Are copies of such documents kept in the library or elsewhere for reference?

How often do you actually receive central guidance? The health service employs over 1 million individuals based at a wide range of varied locations. The problem of sending copies to the right people at the right time is a difficult one to solve. This has eased somewhat

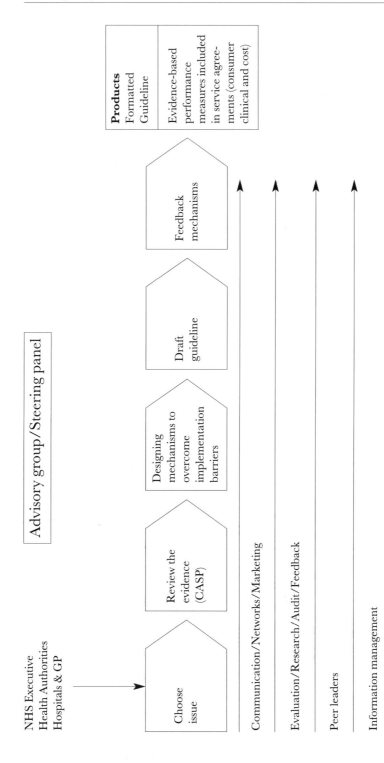

Figure 2.1. Generic model for guideline development and implementation.

with the creation of the Department of Health website, where all centrally produced documents can be accessed, but of course easy access to a computer is necessary and you have to know that the document exists in the first place before you can access it.

The reasons why people do not use evidence are many and varied and, in order for any change to take place, there has to be some value to the person required to make the change. Therefore simply sending out guidelines does not work (Oxman et al., 1995) Other research (NHS Executive, 1993) has shown that a top-down approach will not work either. Any changes based on evidence require teams of health professionals who want to change and have the necessary resources to accomplish the change. For example, evidence-based diabetic guidelines (Hurwitz, Goodman and Yudkin, 1993) recommend the routine screening of large numbers of people. In practice, this creates difficulties for most health authorities because of the amount of resources needed to implement the change.

The development of healthcare quality policy

If we look at quality policy within the NHS over the last decade, we can see that an enormous amount of policy work has taken place recently in an attempt to improve UK health care.

As described in Chapter 1, the process started in January 1989 with the issuing of a White Paper (Department of Health, 1989) and later in Working Paper 6 (Secretaries of State for Social Services, 1989). This made clear the requirement for all doctors and, later, many other health professionals to take part in clinical audit. Audit was well researched and evaluated by several large national studies funded by the Department of Health, and is described and discussed in more detail in Chapter 1. As audit cannot be separated from quality policy, within which it forms an integral part, it is important to recognise that audit itself is not a quality approach. Rather, it is but one tool available to assist us with the implementation of other quality approaches which are outlined below.

Total quality management

Total quality management (TQM) came originally from Japanese economic management. The Department of Health invested a significant amount of resources in 23 national TQM sites throughout the NHS in the early 1990s (Joss, Kogan and Henkel, 1994). The pilots were part funded to introduce a managed approach to quality. The results of the experiment produced six key factors, which need to be in place if successful implementation was to be achieved:

1. Clear management commitment
2. Professional support
3. Designing the service around its customers
4. Developing an organisational framework and system for measurement and improvement
5. Effective communications
6. Actively involving all staff.

Total quality management is a philosophy and way of life and not a simple bolt-on extra. It requires a total cultural change, resulting in continuous improvement, and is an endless process (Figure 2.2).

Regular review and continuous improvement depend as much on attitudes, beliefs and values as they do on actions
Quality in Action – Trafford Health Unit a case study, NHS Management Executive and NHSTD (1993)

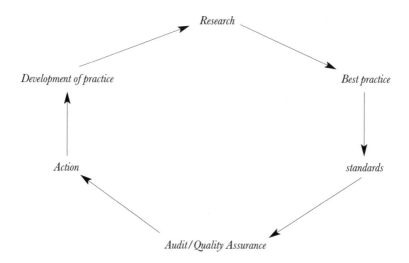

Figure 2.2. Total quality management (TQM) quality cycle. (From Working for You-Hull and Holderness Community Health NHS Trust.

The Patient's Charter

The Patient's Charter (Department of Health, 1991) attempted to put the patient at the heart of the NHS by setting out the rights of patients and some of the standards of care that they could expect:

- Respect for privacy, dignity, and religious and cultural beliefs
- Arrangements to ensure that everyone, including people with special needs, can use the services
- Information for relatives and friends
- Waiting time for an ambulance service
- Waiting time for initial assessment in the accident and emergency department (A&E)
- Waiting time in outpatient clinics
- Cancellation of operations
- A named qualified nurse, midwife or health visitor for each patient
- Discharge from hospital.

For the first time, the health service attempted to ensure that the service shifted from a staff-centred approach to one that considered the needs of the patient. The Patent's Charter included measurable standards for management practice, thus recognising that clinical services alone cannot deliver a health service, but that effective clinical services depend on a range of supporting systems.

Other approaches to quality introduced by the Department of Health and NHS Executive in the mid-1990s, e.g. Patient Focused Care and Business Process Re-engineering, built on this basic premise that health services should be designed around the needs of the consumer.

Quality framework

At the end of 1993 guidance was issued to the NHS, which attempted to pull together much of this work. EL (93) 110 *Achieving an Organisation Wide Approach to Quality* (NHS Executive Letter, 1993a) contained a framework of all the elements necessary to implement and run a high-quality health service. These elements were drawn from the experiences of the NHS pilot sites in total quality management, the national outpatient and A&E demonstration sites, and the experiences of those in the health service who have implemented clinical audit programmes and accreditation systems.

The Executive letter contained the following advice about clinical audit – purchasers and providers should ensure that clinical audit:

- is professionally led;
- is seen as part of the educational process;
- forms part of routine clinical practice;
- is based on standard setting;
- generates results to improve the outcome of care;
- involves managers in the process and outcome of audit;
- is confidential at the individual patient/clinician level;
- is informed by the views of patients/clients;
- becomes part of routine practice for all healthcare professionals and a normal expectation of those who commission and finance health care.

Organisation-wide quality [EL (93) 110]

An organisation-wide approach to quality will be distinguished by the following common factors, which are relevant to both purchasers and providers:

- commitment to quality and leadership from the chief executive;
- quality forming an integral part of both corporate objectives and individual staff objectives, both reflecting the organisation's business;
- the presence of an organisation-wide quality management programme incorporating training in the use of quality tools and techniques;
- all staff have access to training to enable them to develop and make best use of their skills as part of an effective human resource strategy;
- high-quality care achieved through teamwork and partnership, with integrated working involving every member of the organisation;
- effective communications both within the organisation and between it and bodies, e.g. providers, to inform purchasers of structural changes that affect service provision.

Risk management

By 1994, the concept of risk management was attracting a lot of interest as it became clear that the linking of clinical audit, critical incidents and health and safety matters had a significant impact on the quality of care offered by the NHS. Health care is a high-risk business and indeed some risk is essential for continued development. However, it is important that risk-taking is based on sound information and calculated risks and does not occur by accident or poor design. It is extremely important to recognise that most clinical negligence is caused by the failure of the health-care system and not the individual. This means that the NHS still requires a massive cultural shift away from a 'blame' environment to one where mistakes can be admitted and learned from. It also means that those units that implement good quality systems have far fewer critical incidents than those that do not.

In 1993, the NHS Executive had funded two national pilot sites to inform a manual on risk management, which was issued under cover of another Executive Letter EL (93) 111 (NHS Executive Letter, 1993b) to the NHS. The manual gave an assessment of the value of risk management to the NHS, focusing on the cost of poor quality, and identifying quality improvements and the financial benefits flowing from having a risk management policy in place. It gave guidance on the issues to be covered by a risk management survey, and an outline of the principles of risk identification analysis and control. Finally, it contained information about how to monitor systems effectively to ensure that risks were kept under control.

The NHS Litigation Authority manages the Clinical Negligence Scheme for Trusts, which supplies financial incentives for better quality healthcare by means of discounts for NHS hospitals with good risk management schemes. This is intended to reduce the £2 million currently wasted each year in litigation costs, not to mention the enormous cost in terms of human suffering

Business process re-engineering

Around this time, the NHS Executive became aware that more radical approaches towards the implementation of quality approaches were developing in the UK. Several NHS Chief Executives became interested in business process re-engineering (BPR). This built on the principles of other quality approaches, such as total quality management and continuous quality improvement, but was far more radical, requiring the 'fundamental and radical re-design of services around the patient' (Leicester Royal Infirmary, 1994). Business process re-engineering is a short-term but very intensive approach towards improving quality, which if implemented successfully can have dramatic results.

Although it had been tried in American healthcare, by 1994 it was not in use within the UK. The NHS Executive funded two national pilot sites as experimental units from which the rest of the NHS could learn. Developed from industry, BPR is not an easy concept to understand or implement. It requires the massive injection of resources initially and, because it eliminates duplication and waste, it is likely to result in cost savings and efficiencies through the development of services that are very different from those originally in place. Thus, such things as the multiskilling of workforces, redundancies and completely new jobs are common. One example of this was seen in Leicester Royal Infirmary, a national pilot site, where enormous delays were experienced by clinics accessing test results. This problem was solved by making the test results available in one hour, after the creation of a near patient testing site within the outpatient department, staffed by multiskilled health professionals who were able to take blood, radiographs and other tests.

There are a number of key factors necessary for the successful implementation of BPR:

- top level management commitment;
- communication;
- clinical leadership;
- adequate resources.

Re-engineering is not a quick fix and cannot be implemented without the involvement of the entire organisation. Even a whole hospital cannot re-engineer in isolation, because its success or failure depends on the external environment as well as what happens within its internal environment.

Although the national pilot sites produced some interesting results, which included dramatic improvements in service quality, the spread of knowledge throughout the health service has not been so successful. Delays in outpatient clinics, which have been virtually eliminated in the national pilots, are still widespread throughout the rest of the NHS.

> **Challenge**: From the discussion above, which aspects can you identify within your trust? Consider what issues within your speciality are most problematic with regard to risk management. If you were to start with a blank sheet of paper, how could service delivery be re-designed to overcome current problems?

Health policy: the broader context

With the development of commissioning in 1993, when health authorities were created to purchase care on behalf of their populations, improving the quality of care became even more complex. Let us have a look at some of the issues that we need to take into account.

Having a healthy population depends on far more than having effective hospitals and includes a range of factors based around how we live our lives – diet, physical activity, sexual behaviour, smoking, alcohol and drugs. Social and economic issues also have a significant impact – poverty, unemployment and social exclusion – as do environmental factors such as air and water quality and the quality of our housing. Access to services such as education, transport, social services and the NHS itself are important and at the moment are still not equitable to all in the UK. With the Green Paper *Our Healthier Nation* (Department of Health, 1997b; 1998c), the Government actively recognised that policies to improve the nation's health have to be multisectoral and link all of the above elements, e.g. welfare to work, crime, housing and education, as well as health. This is considered in the context of partnerships in Chapter 5. Health authorities have a major part to play in leading these 'health alliances' by developing health improvement plans, which assess local requirements and translate national targets and standards for local action; these are examined later in the chapter.

Hospitals may not necessarily know what services they should plan to deliver because they are not aware of what is required to improve the health of the local population as a whole. This is the role of the public health departments within the health authority through the collection and analysis of epidemiological data. The role of health authorities has now become far more strategic, with a greater emphasis on the monitoring of effective services and by monitoring the progress of their hospitals and general practice units as required by the Regional Offices of the NHS Executive. This monitoring is against nationally set targets contained in documents such as *The Health of the Nation* (Department of Health, 1992) and more recently *Our Healthier Nation* (Department of Health, 1997b). Health authorities and NHS trusts must in future work more in a spirit of collaboration and cooperation to achieve health care that is appropriate, effective and efficient.

In the early 1990s, the role of evidence-based health care in this picture was relatively undeveloped. It is now clear that effective health services should, whenever possible, be anchored in evidence. However, although we now understand the role of evidence, there are still a number of problems to bear in mind when considering the effect of this particular policy decision:

- Although there is a national research and development (R&D) programme, the health service still has a massive lag in terms of the production of evidence of effectiveness for a number of interventions. The time lag between the development of this evidence and its implementation is slow. Examples of the effective management of heart disease, e.g. the use of aspirin as a preventive measure for myocardial infarction, have taken up to 15 years to filter into practice.

- We also have to bear in mind that most evidence is produced and collated by the medical or professional fraternity, assessing issues of a more clinical nature. It is important also to produce economic and consumer evidence to review alongside clinical evidence, i.e. a treatment might be highly effective clinically but its impact on an individual patient, for reasons of either lifestyle or side effects, may make that intervention ineffective for that particular patient.

- Conversely, most evidence is produced by gathering data from large populations, the single-case study approach being regarded as less robust (see Chapter 3). Thus, although an intervention may be highly effective for one individual, the cumulative experiences of a population may prevent that individual receiving appropriate care. An example of this is the operation of tonsillectomy, where the evidence for performing this operation in the vast majority of cases is poor. However, in individuals presenting with a certain set of criteria, the operation is highly effective, dramatically improving the individual's quality of life and saving substantial treatment costs.

• It is also important to consider local factors, e.g. the use of routine ultrasonography in pregnant woman was queried in a 1993 study (Bucher and Schmidt, 1993). However, the study sample was not drawn from a high-risk population, whereas the UK has one of the highest rates of teenage pregnancy in Europe and some severe socioeconomic deprivation in its inner cities, resulting in a higher than normal risk for populations in these groups. Thus, the wholesale implementation of evidence needs very careful thought and the R&D policy centrally has begun to change with the launch of the 1997 White Paper *The New NHS* (Department of Health, 1997a) This set out radical changes to the NHS, including abolishing the internal market and the establishment of primary care groups

The new agenda

In the White Paper, the Department of Health expressed for the first time the wish to slow down the pace of change and looked at the planned introduction of further change over a 10-year time scale. Six main principles underpin the changes:

1. Ensuring that the NHS is a genuinely national organisation.
2. Making the delivery of health care against national standards a matter of local responsibility.
3. Getting the NHS to work together in partnership with local authorities.
4. Driving efficiency by a more rigorous approach to performance and reducing bureaucracy.
5. Encouraging a focus on the quality of care so that excellence becomes the norm.
6. Rebuilding public confidence in the NHS.

This represents a remarkable shift in the development of health policy. The White Paper pulls together many seemingly disparate initiatives, building on earlier work and experience. It promotes the use of national standards and guidelines through:

- the use of evidence-based National Service Frameworks
- the new National Institute for Clinical Excellence (NICE).

These will be supported in their delivery by a range of new organisational mechanisms:

- primary care groups;
- explicit standards in long-term service agreements which replace annual contracts between health authorities, NHS trusts and primary care groups;
- the development of clinical governance systems;
- a new Commission for Health Improvement which will help overcome problem areas.

Again, for the first time, the 1997 NHS White Paper (DoH, 1997) attempts to align financial and other incentives, e.g. the use of non-recurrent cash to reward good performers. The previous system had many perverse incentives, e.g. those hospitals that failed to reduce their waiting lists were given extra money, leaving little incentive to improve spontaneously.

The document *A First Class Service – Quality in the new NHS* (Department of Health, 1998a; Secretary of State for Health, 1998) gives greater detail about how these policy changes are to be implemented and we now look at some of these in detail.

National Service Framework

A new approach to measuring the way the NHS delivers its service is being created. The new National Service Framework (Department of Health, 1998b) replaces the former Purchaser Efficiency index and looks at the quality of care provided by measuring key indicators, rather than at throughput as before. Indicators will be drawn from the following areas:

- patient experiences;
- access to services;
- quality;

- outcome of care;
- health improvement;
- efficiency gain.

The National Service Frameworks build on existing experience such as that gained from the Calman-Hine Report (NHS Executive letter, 1995). They set out what patients can expect in a number of major care areas and diseases. Those currently being worked on include:

- coronary heart disease;
- mental health;
- children's intensive care;
- Calman–Hine cancer services.

Based on evidence of effective practice from a consumer, clinical and cost perspective, these frameworks provide a robust basis for the design, implementation and monitoring of health services.

The National Institute for Clinical Excellence

As stated earlier, NICE is a special health authority with access to a broad range of clinical professionals, NHS managers, and patient and user representatives. Its aim is to ensure that all clinical interventions are embedded in research evidence and to produce detailed guidance for use by both NHS professionals and patients alike. NICE will actually examine the evidence base for all interventions on a priority basis, by using universities to evaluate current research and to scan the horizon for new and potential new developments, which will also be evaluated. The evaluations will be carried out from a cost, clinical and consumer perspective because all three elements are of equal importance in considering whether or not a particular intervention is effective. The sole aim of NICE will be to raise NHS standards, and it will play a major role in ensuring that research evidence passes quickly into practice.

The functions of NICE will be the following:

- to provide guidance to the NHS on: clinical effectiveness, cost-effectiveness and clinical audit methods;

- to appraise new and existing technologies, and develop clinical guidelines for health professionals, patients and carers;
- to produce audit methodologies.

Clinical effectiveness will be both absolute in relation to treatment and relative in relation to current best practice. Cost-effectiveness means that both direct and indirect costs and savings to the NHS, and possibly wider services, will be looked at. Appraisal will look at pharmaceuticals, devices, diagnostics and procedures.

Clinical guidelines will provide guidance on the clinical management of individual conditions based on reviews of the available evidence, clinical effectiveness and cost-effectiveness. There will be new construction and development by NICE, use of the existing Health Technology Assessment programme and the adoption of existing guidelines.

Clinical governance

The concept of clinical governance has already been examined in Chapter 1. It has been defined by Donaldson (1998), the Chief Medical Officer, as:

> A framework through which NHS organisations are accountable for continuously improving the quality of their services and safeguarding high standards of care by creating an environment in which Clinical excellence in clinical care will flourish.

Clinical governance is not new and, in the same way as clinical audit, it does not replace quality but forms one part of a far broader quality picture. Clinical governance sits alongside corporate governance, which can be defined as a duty of good management and financial control – also a part of the quality picture (see Chapter 1).

The principles of clinical governance are the same as those outlined in earlier quality approaches, such as total quality management and continuous quality improvement:

- excellent leadership;
- an organisational culture that fosters education and evaluation;
- communication;
- team working.

The main change is that quality is given the same priority at a Board level as financial performance, representing a major shift of philosophy for the NHS.

In developing clinical governance, the Government and NHS Executive recognise that learning has to take place at the Executive level. Executive directors need to work with their clinical teams to:

- become aware of clinical issues;
- become advocates for the clinical agendas;
- improve the overall quality of clinical care.

How does clinical governance affect you ?

Clinical governance: a workable definition?

Clinical governance places expectations and responsibilities on individuals and organisations to put into place systems to ensure the delivery of high-quality health care to patients.
It places expectations on individuals for:

- working within explicit standards of professional conduct and performance;
- engaging in continuing professional development;
- working in a way that is consistent with the corporate values and the strategic objectives of the organisation.

It places responsibilities on organisations to support clinical staff by:

- encouraging open debate about corporate values and strategic objectives;
- supporting the development of individuals and multidisciplinary teams;
- providing access to national and local information to enable clinicians to plan their services;
- feeding back data to clinicians about their performance;
- ensuring that mechanisms are in place for patients views to be heard;
- ensuring that planned change happens;
- helping clinicians to take action when standards fall below agreed levels.

Health Action Zones

The purpose of the Health Action Zones (HAZs) is:

> To target a special effort on a number of areas where we believe the health of local people can be improved by better integrated arrangements for treatment and care.
>
>   Frank Dobson, The Secretary of State for Health (NHS Executive, 1998)

They have three main objectives:

1. to assess the public health needs of a local area;
2. to increase the effectiveness, efficiency and responsiveness of services, in particular to reduce inequalities in health;
3. to develop partnerships to improve health and services between different agencies.

Health Action Zones involve local authorities, community groups, the voluntary sector and local businesses. They are set up to deliver improvements in health and outcomes, which can be measured and sustained over a long time span. They aim to change local environments by using the enthusiasm and ideas of local people. Again not new, the concept recognises the success of earlier ideas such as the 'Healthy Cities Initiative' and other community programmes that help tackle some of the fundamental causes of ill health.

Primary care groups

There are now approximately 500 primary care groups in the UK. There are four levels of group, which reflect different levels of independence.

Primary care group levels of responsibility (Figure 2.3, see page 42)

Primary care groups bring together GPs, primary care and community nurses, local people, social services, and other healthcare professionals. Primary care groups on levels 1 and 2 will be subcommittees of the health authority, whereas those on levels 3 and 4 will have very little involvement with the health authority. Primary care groups (PCGs) will give primary care a far greater voice in the planning of health systems, eventually resulting in radical change. Their development leaves the NHS with an enormous challenge, as most of those working in primary care are not used to working in large teams or in hierarchical structures. There are many new skills to be developed and many cultural differences to be overcome, as we will see in detail in Chapter 5. Add to this the disillusionment of those enthusiastic fund-holding practices that have now been abolished, and the conversion from the old system to the new is not going to be simple. It is important to remember that the fundamental principles of achieving organisation-wide quality are the same whatever the size or nature of the organisation, so we must not lose sight of the evidence for quality improvement, which can now be applied within PCGs.

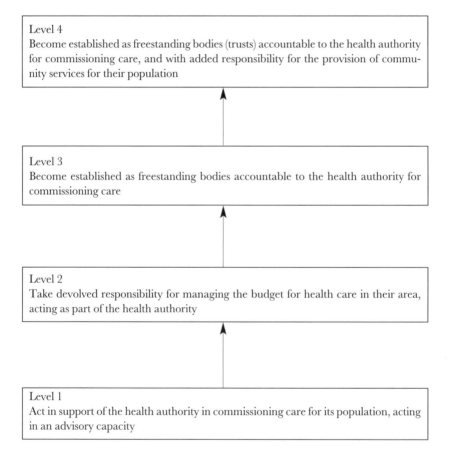

Figure 2.3. Primary care group levels of responsibility.

Not surprisingly, there are as yet few level 3 or 4 PCGs. General practitioners have to be brave to move away from the comfort of the health authority acting as the main agent for commissioning acute and community health-care services.

Health Improvement Plans

Health Improvement Plans are really business plans for health and should encourage all of those working to improve health to work together. Health Improvement Plans will concentrate on three areas: schools and children, workplaces and adults, and neighbourhoods and elderly people. Four priority areas have been identified:

- heart disease and stroke;
- accidents;
- cancer;
- mental health.

If they are linked to the Service Frameworks, address health outcomes and encourage those at health authority, NHS trust and PCG to work together towards common goals, they stand every chance of achieving great success.

Conclusion

Well, how useful is health policy? Without it, we would lack direction and leadership. All those working in the health sector would, in practice, find it very difficult to operate without such guidance. Health policy is influenced by a broad spectrum of views from health professionals, Government, national bodies, and voluntary and other agencies. It is also subject to European and worldwide influences. The most recently developed policies are beginning to be based on evidence of effective practice and to draw on the lessons learned from previous experience from around the world.

References

Black D, Black D, Morris, JN, Smith C (1992) Inequalities in Health – The Black Report. Harmondsworth: Penguin.

Bucher HC, Schmidt JG (1993) Does routine ultra-sound scanning improve outcome in pregnancy? Meta-analysis of various outcome measures. British Medical Journal 307: 13–17.

Department of Health (1989) White Paper. Working for Patients. Cd 555. London: HMSO.

Department of Health (1991) Patient's Charter. London: HMSO.

Department of Health (1992) The Health of the Nation. London: HMSO.

Department of Health (1997a) The New NHS – Modern and Dependable. London: HMSO.

Department of Health (1997b) Our Healthier Nation: A Contract for Health. Cm 3852. London: HMSO.

Department of Health (1998a) First Class Service – Quality in the NHS. London: HMSO.

Department of Health (1998b) National Service Frameworks. London Health Service Circular: HSC 1998/074. London: DoH.

Department of Health (1998c) Our Healthier Nation. London: HMSO.

Donaldson LJ (1998) Clinical governance: a statutory duty for quality improvement. Journal of Epidemiology Community Health 52: 73–4.

Homa P (1994) National Benchmarking Seminar. London: NHS Executive.

Hurwitz B, Goodman C, Yudkin J (1993) Promoting the clinical care of non-insulin dependent (type II) diabetic patients in an inner city area: one model of community care. BMJ (Clinical Research Edition) 1993, March 6; 306. 6878: 624–30.

Joss R, Kogan M, Henkel M (1994) Total Quality Management in the National Health Service: Final Report of an Evaluation. Uxbridge: Centre for Evaluation and Public Policy, Brunel University.

The Leicester Royal Infirmary (1994) Re-engineering the Healthcare Process – Performance Management Framework. Leicester: The Leicester Royal Infirmary.

NHS Executive (1993) The Quality Journey. London: HMSO.

NHS Executive (1998) Health Action Zones – Briefing. NHS Executive 28 BN No 25/27 October 1998. London: NHS Executive.

NHS Executive Letter (1993a) Achieving An Organisational Wide Approach to Quality. EL (93) 110 London: NHS Executive.

NHS Executive Letter (1993b) Risk Management in the NHS. EL (93) 111 London: HMSO.

NHS Executive Letter (1995) A Policy Framework for Commissioning Cancer Services. EL (95) 51 London: HMSO.

Oxman AD, Thomson MA, Davis DA, Hayne RB (1995) No magic bullets: A systematic review of 102 trials of interventions to improve professional practice. Canadian Medical Association Journal 153: 1423–31.

Secretaries of State for Social Services (1989) Working for Patients. Working Paper 6. Cd 555. London: HMSO.

Secretary of State for Health (1998) A First Class Service: Quality in the New NHS. London: HMSO.

Chapter 3
Critical appraisal skills – or don't believe everything you read!

JANE DAWSON

As we have already seen, as for all health-care professionals, nurses are accountable for their practice and are increasingly expected to demonstrate this. This being so, nursing practice should be based on the available research evidence. Clearly, nurses need first of all to know where to look for such evidence and how to make best use of it. A Clinical Standards Advisory Group Report on Stroke Services (Clinical Standards Advisory Group, 1998) found that clinical staff were not skilled in the identification and critical appraisal of research material. Chapter 6 lists the various sources of published research and information on evidence-based practice. What we do in this chapter is to examine how to read and examine that evidence, both at the individual level – research reports and published articles – and at the aggregated level of literature and systematic reviews.

Critiquing an individual research paper

When you decide to look for research evidence on best practice for something in your clinical area, it is not enough simply to find a research report or literature that deals with the subject in which you are interested and blindly set about trying to implement it – and persuade your colleagues to do so as well. You need to be able to appraise a research report or published article critically, in order to decide whether you can have confidence in the findings, and evaluate their appropriateness and relevance to your area of clinical practice.

In this context, the term 'critical' does not mean that the aim is to try to find all the things that are wrong with the piece. It is much more to do with making a balanced and reasoned judgement about the work, rather than accepting that everything that appears in print is bound to be true and flawless. Even in a paper that you decide has flaws, there is almost certain to be something to be learned.

Critical appraisal may sound like something that only nurses in an academic setting can do, but in fact it is a skill that can be learned like any other. Once you learn to read literature in this way, you will find that you get far more out of reading professional books and journals. The key to critical appraisal is to be systematic in your approach. The three main questions you are attempting to answer are:

1. *Why* was the research done?
2. *How* was the study carried out?
3. *What* does it tell you about clinical practice?

Why was the research done?

Look first at the abstract. This should summarise the research and enable you to decide whether it is relevant and applicable to nursing and to your needs. If so, then read on. Is there an introduction and does it identify the research problem that was being addressed? Do *you* consider the problem important? Is it clear what the objectives, aims and hypothesis of the research were? Did the problem arise from the researcher's own work and, if not, why did he or she do this research? This is quite an important point, because it helps to identify whether or not the clinical subject studied was one in which the researcher had considerable experience and the extent of their research experience. Work by someone experienced in research techniques is probably, although not automatically, more reliable than that by a novice researcher. Who funded the research – was it an organisation that would have an interest in a specific result, which would present a potential bias or influence on the research?

How was the research done?

All research needs to be set in the context of previous knowledge on the subject. Is there a literature review that does this? How up to date are the references? If it is an area with which you are familiar, do you feel that the references are appropriate? Do you know of major work that seems to have been omitted? Is the literature discussed and linked logically to the research question? What kind of research design was used – survey, interpretative or experimental, and was this the most appropriate design for the research question? It would, for example, probably be inappropriate to use survey or quantitative techniques to examine the values and beliefs of a small group of patients where there was no previous exploratory work. On the other hand, if the research was to test a new technique, simply asking for the patients' or practitioners' opinion would not be very conclusive!

What was the research setting and/or research sample and how was it selected? You need to look for possible bias and examine the criteria for inclusion or exclusion in the sample of patients studied, such as age, ethnicity or specific symptomatology. If the research setting was unusual or unique, or the sample not really a good representation of the client group, this may have a bearing on how transferable the results are to the clinical setting.

Are the actual methods, e.g. questionnaire or observation, sufficiently described and appropriate to the research question? How were they developed and tested in a pilot study? Is it clear how and by whom the data were analysed? Another point worth considering is whether there are ethical issues with regard to the research. Think what these are and look at whether the paper discusses them and how such issues were handled.

What does it tell you about clinical practice?

First of all, are the results logically presented and related to the research question? Do they meet the original aims and objectives or prove or disprove the hypothesis? Consider whether the conclusion or recommendation is justified by the results, or whether there has been a great conceptual leap without supporting data. Researchers may be at pains to prove their pet theory and ignore or 'reinterpret' inconvenient data! Ask yourself whether alternative explanations or conclusions could have been drawn or better fit the findings. Are there recommendations for future research? Most importantly, what are the implications for clinical practice? Is there evidence to support a change in practice? Consider how the findings match up with current practice in your clinical area, or what would be needed to put any changes into place.

Summary

The purpose of critical appraisal is to form a balanced judgement about the research. It takes practice, but can be learned like any other skill. The checklist below will help you to work through the process logically.

Research problem

Is it clearly set out and its origin explained? Is it amenable to empirical evidence, i.e. can be proved or disproved?

Influencing factors

These include the possible influence of the researchers' background experience, the type of research, the funding body or the supervision, either in conduct of research or in interpretation of results.

Literature review

This should be up to date and comprehensive, and fit well into the research arguments with linked theoretical concepts.

Research objectives and hypothesis

Are these appropriate to the original research question?

Study design

This needs the variables defined, sampling techniques explained and the type of study (experimental, survey or interpretative) clearly set out. Ethical issues have to be discussed and taken into account.

Methodology

This is appropriate to the original question, with explanation of the research tools used and how these were developed, with inclusion of a pilot study and any changes made.

Analysis of data

How is this done and by whom? Have the data been subjected to statistical testing and are the results understandable?

Discussion

The findings need to relate to published research and to the original objectives or hypothesis, with consideration of potential alternative explanations. The limitations of the methods employed are discussed and findings that can be generalised to other populations.

Conclusions and recommendations

Are these justified by the results, do they relate to the original objectives or hypothesis? Recommendations can be made for clinical practice and for further research.

Other aspects

Does the title indicate the subject and is the abstract a succinct summary? Is the paper understandable and well written and are the references accurate?

Research appreciation

Overall, what are your views on the paper? How enjoyable and easy was it to read? The problem is that, as with any other specialised area of knowledge, research has its own language. This language, like any other, is intended to make it easier for meaningful communication to take place, but just like visiting a foreign country it can be difficult for the visitor or newcomer to understand; this may make research seem élitist and research papers full of jargon. Take time to find out and understand what this language means by consulting professional dictionaries and glossaries. Once you become familiar with research terminology, you will see that it does have a purpose. It must be admitted, however, that an abundance of jargon can be used to confuse and provide spurious evidence of expertise. So, if you have problems in gaining even a vague understanding of a research paper, it has failed in its first duty, which is to enlighten the reader.

You will probably find that, once you have learned how to read research critically, you will become much more aware of the potential of nursing literature. Recommendations from research, or even informed discussion of topics related to your clinical speciality, will seem much more relevant and you will be able to make more informed choices as to how these relate to current clinical practice. Kitson (1997a) argues that:

Before you can do the right thing you need to know what the right thing is to do

and that it is important to differentiate between anecdotal reports of practice and rigorous scrutiny of effectiveness. Some people like to have a research awareness file, in which they keep copies of articles of particular interest. One way to do this is to look through relevant journals at regular intervals and pick out those that look interesting for more critical attention. Sometimes libraries offer a research awareness service, or you could join with colleagues to look at a selection of journals and discuss useful items. You could pin important pieces to a noticeboard, located somewhere central such as the coffee room, so everyone can see them.

Alternatively, you could simply keep a card index, or computer database, with references to research papers that you have read and an outline of the contents. That way you can consult your index when a specific topic comes up and refer back to the original source material. Whatever you do, you will find critical appraisal a very useful skill.

Challenge: Look for a research paper relevant to your clinical area. Read it straight through, then write down your immediate views. Now read it again, this time using critical appraisal techniques. Write down your thoughts as you go along. Now compare the two. How different are your notes of the first reading to the appraisal? Did the appraisal change your views on the relevance and applicability of the research to practice? If you can, get a colleague to do the same, and then compare.

Critiquing literature reviews and systematic reviews

Although knowing how to read an individual research paper is a valuable skill, if you were looking for research evidence on which to base your practice, you would undoubtedly want to look at more than one piece of work.

You could go on to carry out your own search of all the literature that you could find related to your topic of interest, and critique and summarise each one in turn using the technique described above, so that you could compare them all at the end. You could even devise a scoring system to rate them. Obviously, this requires access to a wide range of sources and considerable skills in literature searching, not to mention a great deal of time! An alternative is to look for a literature review, in which someone else has searched the literature and evaluated the individual papers, presenting the overall conclusions of research in a particular field. This saves a great deal of time and effort but, as with individual research papers, literature reviews can be conducted for a variety of reasons and vary in their quality and usefulness. The next step is to learn how to appraise a literature review critically.

This is not as daunting as it sounds, but it is not really a task for an inexperienced practitioner who has never undertaken any research or even critiqued a research article. Indeed, Roe (1993) points out that conducting a review of published (and unpublished) research is now a methodology in its own right. A report on research on nursing, midwifery and health visiting (Department of Health, 1993) stated that expert review of research literature is fundamental to the identification of gaps in contemporary knowledge, and went so far as to recommend regular critical reviews of nursing literature. Much has happened since that report, not just in nursing but in all healthcare fields, to put that idea into practice at both a national and an international level, as shown in Chapter 6. Indeed, the whole process of systematic review of healthcare research now receives major government sponsorship and is conducted by units frequently within or closely associated with prestigious university departments.

Nevertheless, if nurses are to play a full part in efforts to make clinical practice evidence-based, they need to be aware of such developments and to gain some knowledge of the processes involved. It is also worth understanding systematic reviews so that individual papers can be set into the context of research literature overall.

In many ways, appraising a literature review is much the same as critiquing an individual piece of work, but on a different scale and in a different context. The first thing to consider in reading a literature review is to ask why it was done. The following are the main reasons for conducting a literature review:

- As part of a research study.
- As an exercise in its own right in order to review current thinking on a particular topic.

- As a tool for summarising, appraising and communicating large amounts of data, in order to determine the weight of evidence for or against a specific intervention in clinical practice.

Although some stages and requirements of a review apply to all three applications, those intended to appraise evidence for specific clinical practice are the most rigorous. Let us look at each of these in turn and see how the requirements, process and purpose differ.

As part of a research study

Literature reviews are a first and continuing activity in conducting a research study. In this case, the purpose of the review is to:

- set the research in context;
- outline current knowledge on the subject;
- review research methods used to explore the subject and support the methods proposed for the current study;
- examine theoretical frameworks or perspectives that underpin past research and/or the current research.

If this is why a literature review has been conducted, it may be useful in updating a practitioner about the current body of knowledge on a subject, and may well provide a shortcut to literature on a topic through the references given. It will, however, have been influenced by the main research question and perspective of the reviewer and directed at his or her requirements. In that case, literature not directly relevant, or which explored alternative arguments, may have been ignored. The review, or an abridged version, will probably be incorporated into the main research report, but if it has been substantial it may well be published as a 'stand-alone' paper.

Challenge: Find an article in a professional journal, or research report, that is related to your clinical area and which contains a literature review. What purpose does the review fulfil? Use the questions listed above on critiquing research papers and apply them to the review. How good do you think the review is? What aspects are good and what are its shortcomings?

As an exercise in its own right to review current thinking on a particular topic

If you have a question related to an area of clinical practice, it is not always necessary to conduct a piece of original research. An alternative approach is to conduct a literature review to find out what research has already been done. Many good research projects are not implemented widely because reports sit on a dusty shelf. McIntosh (1995) wrote of the barriers to implementing research findings and understanding published research was a factor. So, the answer to your question may be out there already if only you look for it!

Another reason for conducting this type of review is to assess the size or prevalence of a problem. This may be to help make a case for a new service, or to demonstrate that a course of action is justified. A literature review can be conducted to justify a proposed research study.

A third reason is simply to update your own professional expertise and knowledge, or that of colleagues. Sometimes a literature review is required to gain acceptance on a degree or other course or as part of a course programme.

This type of review may be purely descriptive, rather than a reasoned critique of the literature covered by the review. The form and medium of publication of the final report will vary according to the circumstances and context in which the review was undertaken.

Challenge: Identify an issue within your clinical area on which you have a question, or where you would like to broaden your knowledge. See if you can find a literature review on the subject or, failing that, a similar area. Apply the techniques described above to see what the purpose of the review was and how well you feel its purpose was achieved.

As a tool for summarising, appraising and communicating large amounts of data in order to determine the weight of evidence for or against a specific intervention in clinical practice.

As has been pointed out earlier, healthcare professionals rarely have the time to identify and read all the research and professional literature available. Just think how many nursing journals there are on the library shelves these days! Systematic reviews are a method of collating large amounts of research material and coming to some overall conclusion. The NHS Centre for Reviews and Dissemination (1996), which is the foremost organisation for this work in the UK, states:

> A systematic review is the process of systematically locating, appraising and synthesising evidence from scientific studies in order to obtain a reliable overview.

This sounds quite complicated and indeed the techniques for carrying out this sort of review are very sophisticated and specialised. It is unlikely that a nurse working in a clinical area would have the facilities, time or expertise to conduct a review of this type. But it is useful to know how they are done and, even more important, how you can judge whether a literature review under-taken for this purpose is useful to your particular situation or prac-tice problem. Literature reviews of this sort are known as systematic reviews.

As the name suggests, systematic reviews are very carefully structured mechanisms, the purpose of which is to evaluate research on the topic under consideration. Broadly speaking, the stages are much the same as for a literature review intended for an individual research study. The key difference is that each stage meets very specific purposes and conforms to carefully defined criteria.

Stages of a systematic review

Stage 1

Systematic reviews are conducted in order to provide information on effectiveness when it is unclear whether a clinical intervention is beneficial or harmful, where clinical practice varies considerably, or when technical changes to the way health care is delivered are proposed or research is planned. So, the first stage is to consider why the review proposed is necessary. The reasons will be documented so that everyone involved knows precisely the purpose of the work. One process, on reaching the decision to proceed, is to identify whether a systematic review on the subject already exists, or is currently being done. There are centres where information on systematic reviews are coordinated, to avoid duplication and provide advice. These are set out and explained in Chapter 6. Another step before work starts is to decide who will be involved. Who are the experts in this field and who will use the findings? Are they willing and able to be part of a group to advise and oversee the work?

Stage 2

The next stage is to look at the boundaries of the review. How much has been written on this subject? What kinds of research have been carried out? The exact questions to be examined by the review must be defined. As the intention is to consider effectiveness of interventions, the measures used to define outcome or benefit must be stated. Is it to be mortality – will it save lives, or are outcomes such as pain relief, less disability and improved quality of life to be considered? If so, the acceptable limits of these must be decided – what is the degree of pain relief achieved by a treatment that will be considered beneficial whereas continued pain above that is considered as evidence that the treatment is non-beneficial? Equally, are there any unwanted side effects that are harmful and how will these be measured? Some of these outcome measures may be indicated by the literature, but precise statements must be made so that consistency is maintained in looking at each research paper on the intervention. Another issue is whether there are factors related to the patient, the way care is delivered or other variables that will influence the effect of the intervention.

All this probably sounds very strange to nurses working on a day-to-day basis with patients, recognising that each one has different needs, that pressures such as the patient's home and family, the need to admit more patients, the availability of a particular drug or service and a host of other variables influence the decisions nurses make from minute to minute. But you have to remember that systematic reviews are intended to make recommendations on practice that are likely to be applicable to the *majority* of patients or health-care settings *overall*. Individual considerations may well override these on a day-to-day basis, but healthcare professionals must make decisions about practice on the basis of knowledge about what is the most likely outcome of a particular intervention, not what is custom and practice for which there is no supporting evidence.

Stage 3

Just as a research study needs a proposal of exactly what is to be done, so a systematic review will have a protocol. The protocol will:

- set out the questions to be answered;
- state how the condition under investigation is to be defined;
- decide what confounding or influencing variables are to be considered, and which patients are to be included and which excluded;
- decide what type of research studies will be reviewed;
- decide what outcome measures will be considered.

Let us look at a specific example. Supposing that the review was planned to consider the evidence on the effectiveness of cardiac rehabilitation after myocardial infarction (MI). The protocol would state for the purpose of the review how the condition of MI was to be defined (suspected or meeting particular cardiac measurements), which patients were to be included (within a certain age band or who only suffered one incident of MI) and what is to be regarded as successful rehabilitation (return to work, ability to walk 2 miles a day), etc. Once these decisions have been made, only research papers that met these criteria would be included in the review. Criteria would also be set for the research itself, such as only randomised control trials, or studies of more than 100 patients over 2 years. In this way, all the research considered will be comparable, so recommendations on effectiveness of the intervention can be made with confidence. The protocol will also state what abstracts, bibliographies and journals will be searched (will it include American or foreign language journals?) and what search terms (key words) will be used, as well as specifying exactly what information will be taken from each article. It would be disastrous, for instance, to review 200 research papers and then realise when you came to write the report that you had forgotten to record the type of rehabilitation programme that each studied!

Stage 4

The next stage in a review is to search and retrieve the literature. This is a major task, but electronic databases such as **MEDLINE, CINAHL, EMBASE** and retrieval mechanisms have made the process much easier than it used to be. There are an increasing number of software programs for managing references – Reference Manager, Idealist – otherwise the search would generate a huge card index that would be very difficult to handle and cross-reference. Once the major abstracts and bibliographies have been searched, other sources should be considered. Conference proceedings can be a useful source and there are databases that record these. There is also the 'grey literature'. This curious term is used to describe internal reports, leaflets, position papers, reviews , etc. by health organisations that have not been published externally in peer-reviewed journals or other mechanisms. Again there are databases for this, but detective work and discussions with experts may identify material. Experts on the subject will be asked to consider the list of literature identified, because they may well have knowledge of other work or sources of information.

Stage 5

Once relevant literature has been retrieved, the studies that they describe need to be assessed. First of all, do they meet the criteria set out in the protocol? If so, the next step is to look at the level of evidence of each. What the level of evidence (sometimes called 'hierarchy of evidence') does is to provide a means whereby studies can be graded according to how strong the evidence that they provide about the intervention really is. There are different models of such hierarchies, but the one in the box is fairly standard.

Level of evidence

1   randomised controlled trials
2a controlled trials with quasi-randomisation
2b controlled trials with no randomisation
3a cohort (prospective) study with concurrent controls
3b cohort (prospective) study with historic controls
3c cohort (retrospective) study with concurrent controls
4   case–control (retrospective) study
5   comparison between times and/or places with and without intervention
6   opinions of respected authorities, clinical experience; descriptive studies; reports of expert committees

---

If you think about different kinds of research design that you might use in a study investigating whether or not an intervention is effective, randomised controlled trials (RCT) will make the strongest case. To find out whether a particular drug has the effect that manufacturers claim, the research is set up so that relevant patients are divided into two groups: one is given the experimental drug and the other is treated in the usual way. Patients are randomly allocated to the two groups so that the chances of being given the experimental drug are the same for every patient in the sample. No-one (patient or doctor) should know which patients are receiving the experimental drug. The outcome (how did it affect patients?) is measured in the same way for all patients and all other possible variables (age, sex, nature of illness) are carefully controlled and taken into account in the analysis. This is clearly much stronger evidence than if you gave a few patients the new drug and asked them if they felt better. Obviously, between these two extremes there are a range of different research designs and what assessment of the level of evidence does is to put them in rank order, from the strongest to the weakest.

The biggest difference is between studies that follow an experimental design (such as RCTs and similar designs) where the allocation of patients and other variables is carefully controlled, and studies that observe differences between patients, but where treatment choice is more haphazard. It is much harder in the latter to demonstrate that differences in patient outcomes are the result of differences in treatment, not some other variable.

Oddly enough, the lowest level of evidence is that of the expert opinion. You might think that what the experts consider the best way to treat a patient is bound to be the best approach, but this is not necessarily the case. Experts can only go on their clinical experience to date and they may not have encountered the experimental drug or treatment under consideration. Experts can and frequently do disagree. Also, even experts may have prejudices and pet theories that would not stand up to scientific examination. However, where clear evidence is equivocal or does not exist, expert opinion may be the only and best option for reaching a recommendation and is certainly better than leaving every single practitioner to make up his or her own mind.

In considering the quality of the review, one factor is the strength of the evidence of the studies included. A review that only covered reports based on expert opinion alone would be less reliable than one in which a number of RCTs or good observational studies had been considered.

Stage 6

The data collection as set out in the protocol will then be conducted. As for all good research, the kinds of data will depend on the questions the review is intended to answer. Data extraction forms will be designed and pilot testing carried out on a number of reviews. If the review is being done by more than one person, then cross-checking for compatibility and consistency is necessary. Decisions need to be made on what to do where data are missing or incomplete. Sometimes, it may be necessary to recalculate the data where the information is not presented in a way that meets the requirements of the review, e.g. if patients in a subgroup are given in numbers, not percentages, or no totals given. This must be done with caution, however, so as not to cause distortions, and will require the advice of a statistician. It may be difficult to follow the detail of this stage, but it should conform to the agreed protocol and explanations be given on missing data, reliability between reviewers and so on.

Stage 7

Data synthesis is required to come to an overall conclusion. If this is not done, all you have is an uncritical description of the literature. A review should give an estimate of the average effect of the intervention under study, show whether and by how much this varies between studies, and consider why such differences may have arisen. Data collation or synthesis is a highly specialised technique, requiring complex statistical calculations that few nurses are likely to understand, but the review should contain a narrative that sets out the overall conclusions clearly.

Stage 8

The report is of course the final phase in the review. In many ways the contents will be similar to those of a report on a research study and will contain the following:

- An abstract or summary that provides an outline of each individual section.
- An outline of the background and need for the review. This will describe the original health-care dilemma and the clinical situation and professionals to which the report is relevant.
- The hypothesis and research questions addressed.
- The methods employed, including the search strategy, how data were extracted and analysed.
- A detailed description of studies included in the review and also of those excluded, with reasons for this.
- The overall results, which will consist mostly of statistical tables and confidence intervals and may well include tests of the strength of findings.
- A discussion of the study itself, possible biases, limitations, etc.
- The implications of the findings for clinical practice. By the very nature of systematic reviews, this will be related to populations or groups of patients, e.g. all women with breast cancer. However, clinicians are likely to be influenced by findings and consider them when making decisions about the care of an individual patient.

Summary

You can no doubt see that literature reviews and, in particular, systematic reviews are complex undertakings. Consequently, appraising a review is more difficult and requires a lot more time and thought. However, the checklist below will help:

1. Was the subject of the review clear and unambiguous? This should be in terms of the population studied, the intervention and outcomes.
2. Were the studies included suitable? You might consider whether they were relevant to the main review questions and their design appropriate.
    If the answer to both these questions is 'No', then it may not be useful to continue.
3. How good was the search for useful literature? Look at which bibliographic databases were used, and whether 'grey literature' was included, experts personally consulted, non-English language studies included.

4. How careful were the authors to evaluate the quality of the studies included? Think about the hierarchy of evidence that we looked at earlier.
5. Was combination of study results justified? As explained earlier, sometimes study results are combined and recalculated. If this was done, were studies similar enough in conduct and findings to make this a sensible step?
   If the answer to these questions is 'Yes', the methodology of the review was good.
6. What are the results? Is it clear what the reviewers are saying about the intervention studied? How are these set out?
7. How exact are the figures? Confidence limits (a statistical test of reliability) will be presented in major reviews.
   These last two questions should make it clear what the results actually were.
8. Will the findings be helpful locally? Are there important differences between local patients and settings and those in the review studies?
9. Were the outcomes considered in the review important? Were others omitted?
10. Does the benefit outweigh the possible harm and cost? A good review will include this, but, if not, what do you think?

However good the review, there may be factors that make it inappropriate to introduce the findings locally
   You can no doubt see that undertaking a systematic review, or assessing the quality of one is not something that most nurses will either wish, or have the need, to do. It is sometimes argued (Kitson, 1997b), that the scientific basis for nursing is still relatively undeveloped, and that the very nature of much nursing makes carefully controlled experimental studies inappropriate (Naish, 1997). This latter point is now being addressed with efforts to identify RCTs in nursing (Droogan and Song, 1996; Cullum, 1997). However, if nurses are to take responsibility for ensuring that their own clinical practice is effective, as well as playing an increasing part in the healthcare team in decision-making, they need to develop some understanding now of the mechanisms by which research evidence is assessed and recommendations for practice made.

References

Clinical Standards Advisory Group (1998) Report on Clinical Effectiveness Using Stroke Care as an Example. London: HMSO.

Cullum N (1997) Identification and analysis of randomised controlled trials in nursing: a preliminary study. Quality in Health Care 6: 2–6.

Department of Health (1993) Report of the Taskforce on Strategy for Research in Nursing, Midwifery and Health Visiting. London: HMSO.

Droogan J, Song F (1996) A Review of Systematic Reviews in Nursing. Newcastle: National RCN Research Conference.

Kitson A (1997a) Doing the right thing right. Nursing Practice 9(1): 16–19.

Kitson A (1997b) Using evidence to demonstrate the value of nursing. Nursing Standard 11(28): 34–9.

McIntosh J (1995) Barriers to research implementation. Nurse Researcher 2(4): 83–90.

Naish J (1997) So where's the evidence? Nursing Times 3(12): 64–6 .

NHS Centre for Reviews and Dissemination (1996) Undertaking Systematic Reviews of Research on Effectiveness. CRD Report 4. University of York.

Roe B (1993) Undertaking a critical review of the literature. Nurse Researcher 1(1): 31–41.

Chapter 4
The role of education in supporting clinically effective practice

Sue Torkington

No debate about clinical effectiveness would be complete without a discussion on the role of education in supporting effective practice. Moores and Jarrold (1994) consider that effective education and training are the bedrock of professional practice, which aims to provide the highest standards of care for patients and clients, their families and the wider community.

Health professional education is itself required to be effective, responsive, appropriate and accountable. The aim of health professional education is to equip clinicians with theoretical and practical knowledge, clinical skills and professional attitudes to enable them to be fit for practice, fit for purpose and fit for academic award. To achieve these outcomes, educational experiences and learning opportunities have to be relevant to the strategic direction of the health service, to the health needs and priorities of people who use the service, and to the business plans and resources of service providers.

Here we take an educational perspective on issues discussed in other chapters. We will explore ways in which education providers can participate in initiatives that support clinically effective interventions and evidence-based practice, first, by considering the relationship between education and clinical effectiveness and, second, by reviewing educational opportunities and resources that support the promotion of clinical effectiveness. A case study and scenario are used to illustrate the ideas and issues raised.

The relationship between nursing education and clinical effectiveness

Policy changes in the NHS, such as clinical governance (Department of Health, 1998a), are creating new relationships between education and practice. As change is a continuous feature of modern healthcare, it is essential that educational initiatives and provision are responsive and flexible to meet the needs of nursing students, practitioners and managers. Humphreys (1996) suggests that education and training need to be seen as a strategic issue – that is to say highly significant in terms of organisational development, particularly in the context of NHS reform. In a similar review, Corbett (1998) concludes that the NHS needs nursing education to support enhancement of services, whereas the United Kingdom Central Council (UKCC, 1992b) reports that changing health needs require nurses to re-skill.

Maynard (1988) suggests that, historically, millions of pounds have been spent on care provided on the basis of value judgements and hope, rather than on proven research evidence. This view is supported by Dunn et al. (1997) who conclude that in the past the majority of healthcare has been largely based on opinion rather than on evidence of clinical effectiveness. Walshe and Ford (1995) observe that ritualistic nursing practices can still be found, a situation perhaps explained by Regan's (1998) observation that not all nurses currently practising have been educated in such a way as to equip them with the necessary skills to evaluate research critically – a prerequisite for evidence-based care. This appears to support Humphreys' (1996) argument that new nurses need to differ from old nurses in various ways.

Changing practice to reflect evidence and demonstrate the effectiveness of care is a complex activity and requires the development of a particular range of skills. This challenge is reflected in the Government Green Paper *Our Healthier Nation* (Department of Health, 1998b), which highlights the need to equip nurses with the skills and knowledge required to achieve greater involvement in the public health agenda and to demonstrate the clinical effectiveness of nursing. Providing evidence of the clinical effectiveness of nursing interventions will help to demonstrate the value and expertise of nursing both to the client and to the NHS.

McClarey (1998) notes that, in spite of convincing arguments, numerous projects and the existence of considerable information, clinically effective practice is still not being widely implemented. Swage (1998) reflects that one of the current problems of implementing evidenced-based care may be the result of nurses' lack of knowledge about what clinical effectiveness means in theory and practice. However, the complexity of changing professional behaviour is well documented in the literature and spans all health-care professional groups. Walshe and Ham (1997) believe that there has been an apparent lack of concern and debate about clinical effectiveness by senior management and this is reflected in the practice of clinicians. This has been acknowledged and is being addressed through requirements in the White Paper *The New NHS* (Department of Health, 1998a), which gives all health organisations a statutory duty to seek quality improvements.

Swage (1998) observes that the White Paper makes it clear that clinical governance places a duty on all health professionals to ensure that care is satisfactory, consistent and responsive. In addition, under the arrangements for clinical governance, nurses will have to take part in continuing professional development. Clinical governance has been defined by Scally and Donaldson (1998) as a system through which NHS organisations are accountable for continuously improving the quality of their services and safeguarding high standards of care by creating an environment in which clinical care will flourish. A number of new initiatives and mechanisms have been put in place (see Chapter 2), which will support education and practice in meeting the requirements of clinical governance. The National Institute of Clinical Excellence has been set up and will promote clinical and cost-effective care by producing research-based guidelines. National service frameworks will set out the patterns and levels of service that should be provided for major care and disease groups (Black, 1998). Recommendations arising from these developments will need to be incorporated into practice, and this may require practitioners to change established patterns of behaviour. This will require new approaches to education and training, such as problem-based learning, the development of critical appraisal skills and the reorientation of staff to manage rapid change.

The development of education consortia has given NHS trusts and health authorities direct control over the type of training and education received by large numbers of staff. Consortia emerged from the changes brought into being by Working Paper 10 *Working for Patients* (Department of Health, 1989). Through a process of expanded devolution, consortia have now become commissioners of non-medical education and training, and hold the training budget, variously referred to as non-medical education and training (NMET) or Working Paper 10 money. Elliott and Pickering (1997) report that education consortia are responsible for collating information from local healthcare organisations and turning it into educational contracts that will meet the needs of all the local service providers. This process has the potential to deliver education that is flexible, effective and efficient, and meets the needs of employers and practitioners. However, Humphreys (1996) warns that some consortia have been too focused on operational aspects of educational commissioning rather than on educational outputs, e.g. the skills of the resulting practitioners and the strategically significant relationship between these outputs and the current and future needs of the health service.

Humphreys (1996) reflects that, when a consortium does focus on issues such as the future nature of health services (e.g. clinical governance), the new type of practitioner (e.g. a knowledgeable, questioning doer) and the implications of this for course content and output, it will, through its commissioning role, generate change that will impact on and facilitate changes in practice such as clinically effective care.

Education providers, now mainly universities, need to work closely with purchasing trusts to develop responsive educational provision. Responsive education is part of a quality strategy that meets the education and continuing professional development needs of practitioners working in health services and addresses requirements at both a local and a national level. This may be through working in partnership with clinical staff, service users and researchers to develop new programmes or courses, through the provision of novel course delivery, such as distance or computer-assisted learning, or through the provision of learning resources such as library and information services.

Farmer and Richardson (1997) consider that perhaps the single most important thing that policy-makers could do to encourage evidence-based practice among health professionals is to provide good access to both information professionals and information resources. Walshe and Ham (1997) comment on how few health authorities or trusts provide access to the standard citation databases of nursing and allied health literature, and other commentators express concern about the inequitable access to health libraries since the incorporation of nursing education into academia. This means that access to library and information services for nurses has developed in an isolated and fragmented way (Capel, 1998). Complicated funding arrangements have contributed to the difficulties experienced by many nurses in using libraries. In addition, Fennessy (1998) suggests that nurses are often unaware of existing library facilities and services. As libraries are a basic requirement for access to professional knowledge, there is much discussion in the literature about these concerns and various proposals to address the situation are being explored. For example, the Nursing Standard Libraries Access Campaign in November 1997 helped to raise awareness of the importance of health libraries and information services

Godbolt, Williamson and Wilson (1977) reflect that the move of nurse education into higher education has had a profound impact on library services in both universities and the NHS. Access to university libraries requires the local agreement of consortia, trusts and universities to ensure that suitable arrangements are put in place. A number of contemporary issues complicate this activity, e.g. the development of multimedia resources and increasing professional specialisms have resulted in an expansion of the range and cost of educational materials available. Various academic levels, from certificates to PhDs, require resources that challenge and inform in a relevant way. In addition, research and policy publications need to be available within appropriate time frames and in well-presented formats that can be accessed by a wide audience.

Historically, a lack of attention to these issues may have created some of the difficulties experienced by nurses in accessing published research. The NHS Executive (1998a) notes that clinicians have identified that both out-of-date textbooks and disorganised journals create barriers to obtaining clinically important information. Nurses need accurate, concise reference sources to answer specific patient-oriented questions. Cullum, DiCenso and Ciliska (1998) considers that they need the answer quickly, they need to be able to trust it and it needs to be at their fingertips. Access to a library service that provides appropriate literature and multimedia resources, has flexible opening hours and offers Internet and appropriate database facilities would appear to be an absolute requirement for promoting evidence-based, clinically effective practice.

The NHS Centre for Reviews and Dissemination (1999) proposes that there is a naïve assumption that, when research information is made available, it is accessed by practitioners, appraised and then applied in practice. Ibbotson, Grimshaw and Grant (1998) suggest there is a recognised gap between the publication of research findings and their adoption in practice, a view shared by Hunt (1981), Bircumshaw (1990), and Webb and Mackenzie (1993). The reasons for this continuing problem are multifactorial, but appear to focus on a number of issues such as nurses finding research reports incomprehensible (Camiah, 1997), lack of time to search for information (Ibbotson et al., 1998) or because they lack confidence, as a result of not being taught how to find and appraise research (Pearcey, 1995).

Recognition of these factors, together with the shift from registration for life to creating life-long learners, has resulted in rapid expansion of continuing education opportunities which support both the individual practitioner's need for professional development and the employer's need to develop an appropriate skill base. Elliott and Pickering (1997) consider that the key to staff development is appropriate use of individual performance review, suggesting that individual performance review (IPR) or appraisal is about the employer and employee moving forward together, developing individuals in the performance of their role and meeting corporate objectives, e.g. clinically effective care.

There is little doubt that there is a strong correlation between staff development and the quality of service that they provide. Barriball, While and Norman (1992) argue that one of the fundamental functions of continuing professional education is to enhance the quality of patient care, a view shared by Hogston (1995). Scally and Donaldson (1998) suggest that designing programmes that help to advance the quality goals of every organisation, and that draw on evidence, will be part of the principles of good clinical governance.

The preceding discussion has explored a number of key issues within the clinical effectiveness debate, e.g. clinical governance, education consortium, and access to library and information services. The following case study provides an example of how a healthcare trust can begin the process of creating educational opportunities through the contracting process.

Case study 1

Seaside Healthcare Trust commissions nurse education through the Downland Education Consortium. Janet Williams, Director of Nursing Services, represents the Trust on the Consortium, which also supports five other trusts. Two universities provide education via an education contract negotiated by the Consortium. Each year Janet is required to put forward the numbers of nursing students that the Trust wishes to commission in order to meet the Trust's workforce planning needs. These numbers are closely related to the level of service, which the Trust has determined will allow it to meet its strategic plan at the quality standards agreed. The Consortium has a role to play in helping Seaside Trust to collate its workforce plans and estimate demand for newly qualified staff. In 1999, the Trust requested 45 adult nursing students, 30 mental health students and 15 child health students. In addition, the Trust had made a commitment to support 10 enrolled nurses who wished to convert to registered nurses.

Seaside Trust had also negotiated NMET money to develop its qualified staff and had been allocated this in the form of person training days (PTDs). Senior staff from different clinical directorates within the Trust had met with education staff from one of the universities, which provided both pre- and postregistration education, to determine what type of courses, study days and workshops could be developed to meet the continuing professional development needs of their staff. Nurse managers recognised that the education needs of their staff needed to be met in order for them to deliver high-quality, effective care and had established areas of priority through matching IPR/appraisal information with clinical audit data and health-care policy documents. During the discussions, a local agreement was put in place to ensure access to the university library for all nursing staff, not just for those enrolled on university courses.

Educational opportunities and resources that support the promotion of clinical effectiveness

The vision of continuous quality improvement and the introduction of clinical governance rest on a clear commitment to continuing professional development and life-long learning (Department of Health, 1999). The NHS Executive (1998b), in an investigative study of continuing professional development, states categorically that the practice of a health professional carries an obligation to life-long learning. Various healthcare policies, reports and stated professional priorities indicate that life-long learning and continuing professional development are the responsibility of individual practitioners, professional bodies and employers, within both the NHS and the private sector.

These obligations are explicit in *The Code of Professional Conduct* (UKCC, 1992a), which states that each nurse is responsible for improving professional knowledge and competence. Similarly, *The Scope of Professional Practice* (UKCC, 1992b) sanctions nursing practice based on independent judgement and sound principles. These statements are supported by recommendations contained in the Post-Registration Education and Practice (PREPP) document *The Future of Professional Practice: The Council's Standards for Education and Practice Following Registration* (UKCC, 1994). However, the document *A Vision for the Future* (Department of Health, 1993) acknowledges that professional bodies must also ensure that the educational needs of nurses and midwives are met in order for them to deliver high-quality care.

In Working Paper 10, *Working for Patients: Education and Training* (Department of Health, 1989), there is an emphasis on the responsibility of the direct employer for training and education. These priorities are also reflected in the Audit Commission report (1991), which states that good quality nursing care requires not only that the staffing of wards is adequate but also that nurses are equipped with the right skills and education to adapt to modern care requirements. The document *The New NHS – Working Together: Securing a Quality Workforce for the NHS* (Department of Health, 1998a) commits NHS organisations to supporting continuing professional development through the introduction of personal development plans that are linked to performance appraisal and organisational objectives.

Continuing professional development (CPD) or education (CPE) has been variously defined. The American Nurses' Association (1984) considers that CPD is any planned activity intended to build on the educational and experiential bases of the professional nurse, for the enhancement of practice, education, administration, research or theory development, to the end of improving the health of the public. The English National Board (ENB, 1990) suggests that CPE is any post-basic education, which is directed at maintaining and improving the quality of care provided to the public. CPE is endorsed by the UKCC (1990) as the chosen method for maintaining professional knowledge and competence.

There appears to be consensus in the literature that well-targeted CPE promotes more effective practices (Davis et al., 1995; Hogston, 1995; Furze and Pearcey, 1999). However, changing practice to reflect evidence and demonstrate the effectiveness of care is a complex activity and requires multifaceted educational approaches and experiences.

Although the NHS invests major resources into CPD, the NHS Executive (1998b) is concerned at the lack of research-based evaluation of CPD. The NHS Executive (1998b) also challenges the methodological adequacy of some research and requests more descriptive and comparative studies of both traditional and innovative evidence-based educational programmes. Fitzpatrick, While and Roberts (1994) suggest that measuring the quality of education is always problematic partly as a result of the difficulty of obtaining evidence on the performance of trained nurse output. However, there is evidence to support the argument that well-qualified and experienced nurses have a positive impact on cost-effective and clinically effective care (Aiken, Smith and Lake, 1994; Brown and Grimes, 1995; Griffiths, 1996). A number of rigorous evaluation studies of continuing medical education (CME) are available and, with the growing trend towards multidisciplinary education, it seems appropriate to include a small sample to inform the debate.

In a comprehensive review, Davis et al. (1995) identified 99 studies involving 160 comparisons of CME interventions, including the following:

• educational materials;

- formal CME programmes such as conferences, seminars, work-shops;
- educational outreach (visits by educators or clinical specialists);
- local opinion leaders.

Results indicated that, although single interventions were likely to be effective, multifaceted interventions, which also assessed potential barriers to change, were likely to be more successful.

In a similar study, Oxman et al. (1995) found that there was a wide range of educational interventions which, if used appropriately, could lead to important improvements in professional practice and patient outcomes. Oxman et al. identified that dissemination-only strategies such as conferences demonstrated very little or no change in health professional behaviour or health outcome when used alone. Likewise, Smith (1998) conceded that there are no hard data to demonstrate that academic journals have any effect in promoting evidenced-based practice. Oxman et al. (1995) concluded that there are no 'magic bullets' for improving the quality of healthcare, but there is a wide range of interventions available which, if used appropriately, could lead to substantial improvements in clinical care.

Waddell (1991) found that continuing education affects nursing practice positively, reporting that there was a greater likelihood of effect when learners were from the same practice environment and planned their continuing education activities accordingly. Similar results are recorded by Nolan, Owens and Nolan (1995), Jordan and Hughes (1998) and Wildman et al. (1999). For additional examples, the *Effective Health Care Bulletin* (NHS Centre for Reviews and Dissemination, 1999) gives a comprehensive review of other studies and provides a range of helpful and relevant advice to those involved in changing practice.

The bulletin also proposes that, if the current goal to improve clinical effectiveness is to be achieved, it is essential that there are mechanisms by which individual and organisational change can occur. It is widely accepted in the literature that, although individual beliefs, attitudes and knowledge influence professional behaviour, organisational factors are also important. This has been illuminated in Barriball and While's (1996) study, which considers participation in CPE in nursing. Barriball and While (1996, p. 1006) conclude that:

> Poor funding, low staffing levels and domestic responsibility will deter practi-
> tioners' participation in continuing professional education unless careful
> consideration is given to CPE in terms of scheduling, location and funding as
> well as its quality and relevance to the professional and personal development of
> practitioners.

Funding for CPE is recognised as being inequitable by a number of writers, e.g. Furze and Pearcey (1999), Hogston (1995) and Nolan et al. (1995), and this is being acknowledged as a problem in a number of reports (e.g. Audit Commission, 1991). The document *Making a Difference* (Department of Health, 1999) also addresses issues, such as low staffing levels and the need for employment flexibility for practitioners with domestic responsibility.

The issue of relevance to the professional and personal development of practitioners is explored by Scheller (1993), who suggests that it is important for educators to consider the potential impact and effectiveness of continuing education during programme or course development. Considering the factors that will influence nurses' use of knowledge gained from a learning experience, and addressing the issues raised, will ultimately contribute to the implementation of clinically effective care. Scheller discovered a number of recurring themes, which illustrated factors that prevented nurses making use of the knowledge that they had acquired. The first theme was nurses' perceived inability to make the application of knowledge from continuing education a priority in their clinical area. Various explanations were offered, such as:

• inadequate time for thoughtful incorporation of knowledge into practice;
• the stresses of job demands;
• no reinforcement to make the application of continuing education knowledge a priority.

The second theme that emerged in Scheller's (1993) study was resistance to change. It seems incomprehensible that nurses who express a commitment to clinical effectiveness and evidence-based practice should resist opportunities to change practice after professional development. However, critical issues surrounding the use of new knowledge in practice included the following:

- perceived lack of control in relation to change;
- reactions to strong informal group leaders who respond negatively to change;
- the perception that the proposed change threatens the values of the group.

Humphreys (1996) argues that continuing education provision should, among other things, help to reorientate staff in the context of planned change and help with skill mix; this creates an additional role for education in relation to clinical effectiveness. In addition, Humphreys perceives that there is a need to match educational outcomes with health outcomes, and to overcome traditional nursing hierarchies.

Scheller (1993) drew a number of interesting conclusions from her research, including the observation that nurses will not use CPE knowledge that they perceive as threatening to their control of nursing and the values surrounding their nursing practice. This statement raises an important issue about nursing knowledge and the value systems from which it develops. Kenny (1997) asserts that, within the medical profession, knowledge is commonly interpreted as a matter that can be verified by the scientific, biomedical method (e.g. randomised controlled trials). However, Kenny (1997) also acknowledges that this traditional medical epistemology fails to represent medical knowledge adequately, because human interpretation cannot be investigated from this position. Nurses have been concerned about investigating and interpreting the art and science of nursing for a number of years. Carper (1978) identified four sources of nursing knowledge, including:

- scientific or empirical evidence;
- personal and moral knowledge;
- aesthetics or art of nursing.

These perspectives create a tension between using qualitative and using quantitative research methods to inform evidence-based practice and clinical effectiveness in nursing.

Currently, the NHS Executive (1996) stated preference is for the evaluation of all health-care interventions to be actioned through randomised controlled trials and these form the basis of the

Cochrane Centre Database. This directive will undoubtedly restrict the participation and contribution of nurses to the debate, and much valuable and important clinical and patient/client evidence could be lost. Kitson (1997) proposes that the evidence-based practice and clinical effectiveness movements have to acknowledge the characteristics of nursing. This calls for a broader methodological base on which to evaluate evidence and clinical effectiveness, which will require wider definitions for diagnosis and treatment and more interest and investment in non-pharmacological interventions.

The ability to contribute to these types of professional debate requires clinicians and practitioners to have confidence in dealing with conflicting ideas, and ambiguity and competence in recognising the validity and applicability of research evidence. Swage (1998) reflects that many nurses are not confident in relation to their understanding of research and reviews; however, it is interesting to note that this also appears to be a problem for other healthcare professionals. In response to these concerns, Oxford and Anglia Region instituted a clinical appraisal skills programme (CASP) as part of getting research into its practice and purchasing programme, with the aim of helping decision-makers to develop skills in the critical appraisal of evidence about effectiveness (Houghton, 1997). Research into critical appraisal has indicated that doctors trained in critical appraisal skills as undergraduates retain those skills and remain more clinically competent and up to date than those trained by more traditional methods (Sackett and Rosenberg, 1995). McClarey (1998) develops these findings by proposing that educational programmes can promote clinical effectiveness in nursing through ensuring that both pre- and post-registration nurses have critical appraisal skills (see Chapter 3). The latter should equip nurses to remain clinically competent throughout their careers by enabling them to seek, assess and make use of up-to-date knowledge to inform their decision-making in practice.

The preceding debate has raised a number of issues, which are relevant and important when identifying educational opportunities and resources that support the promotion of clinical effectiveness. The responsibility of individual practitioners, professional bodies and employers has been considered, and various reports and documents have been reviewed. The definition and scope of continuing education have been explored and research evidence relating to a variety of continuing education interventions and opportunities has been examined. The impact of continuing education on nursing practice has been considered and some of the constraints relating to changing practice discussed. It has also been proposed that clinical effectiveness and evidenced-based practice have to be informed by a range of methodological approaches and that nurses need critical appraisal skills in order to manage the complexity of contemporary health-care delivery.

The scenario in the box provides an example in which the issues raised can be illustrated.

Liz Brown and Shirley James work for the Sovereign Community Trust. They are both district nurses who are frequently required to supervise nursing students from Riverside University. Liz has been a district nurse for 20 years, but Shirley only finished her degree in community nursing 9 months ago.

Shirley enjoys having the nursing students; she likes the way that they question her and challenge her. If she does not know the answers to their questions, she is happy to go the library to access online journals to find relevant information and she always seems to be able to refer to the latest policy statement or report. Shirley has requested to go on a leg ulcer management course because she is aware that, with the number of patients on her caseload with leg ulcers, she needs to develop her knowledge base and skills. She has already put together some research information about leg ulcers and has challenged the GP's management of two patients. Shirley was surprised that the GP seemed pleased that she had started to evaluate care so thoroughly, and they have discussed the possibility of writing some clinical guidelines.

Liz finds Shirley a little bit overwhelming, and also finds the students heavy going. She is becoming increasingly worried about being asked questions that she cannot answer and finds that students often talk to her about research that she has never heard of. The university has just appointed a lecturer practitioner (Jenny Clark) to support Sovereign Community Trust staff in practice development. Jenny has a district nurse background with 10 years' practice experience and has achieved a BSc in Nursing Studies and an MSc in Community Practice. When Liz met her she found her approachable and very enthusiastic, so Liz decided to ask for advice about her own professional development needs. Jenny was pleased to help and, after listening to Liz's concerns, suggested that they should do a review of Liz's experience; this proved to be very helpful. Liz had qualified as a registered general nurse in 1970 and during her training had not been encouraged to challenge opinion or debate issues. She had been encouraged to learn by rote what she was told and there had been very little facility to explore the nursing literature or suggest new ideas in practice. Although Liz had a wealth of experience as a district nurse and was regarded as a competent professional, she was aware that she needed to address her lack of confidence in challenging established practices that needed to be reviewed and updated. Liz and Jenny identified that, because Liz had not had the opportunity to engage in any continuing professional development, she was missing out on some important educational opportunities and experiences. Jenny helped Liz develop a professional development plan around her own personal and professional needs, and encouraged her to seek accreditation for her prior experiential learning (APEL).

Liz decided that she would enrol for the first year of a flexible diploma programme at the university. After discussions with the Community Pathway Leader, Liz started with the research awareness course, which was designed to help practitioners question established practice and to explore ways of being more effective through examination and evaluation of the research literature. This gave Liz the opportunity that she needed to develop her thinking and to analyse information and debate issues in a safe, but challenging, environment. She began to engage in constant reflection and appraisal of her nursing interventions and welcomed debate and discussion with her colleagues and nursing students.

Conclusion

Education can provide practitioners with the opportunity to think critically and creatively, with the confidence to challenge and perhaps more importantly to be challenged without feeling threatened or undermined. These are the characteristics of an educated person – the practitioner described by the Project 2000 document as a knowledgeable doer . . . a thinking person with analytical skills. It is becoming increasingly obvious that, with the rate and pace of change in nursing, intellectual cognitive skills as well as clinical psychomotor skills need to be enhanced in order for nurses to address the complexity of contemporary practice.

This chapter has discussed the role of education in supporting clinically effective practice. Through exploration of the key issues, it has become evident that nursing practice and nursing education are both dependent on constant analysis of the purpose and goals of nursing and committed to assessing the outcomes of their interventions. It is an inevitable conclusion that enhancing and demonstrating clinical effectiveness is a joint responsibility.

References

Aiken L, Smith H, Lake E (1994) Lower medicare mortality among a set of hospitals known for good nursing care. Medical Care 32: 771–87.

American Nurses' Association (1984) Standards for Continuing Education in Nursing. Kansas City: American Nurses' Association.

Audit Commission (1991) The Virtue of Patients: Making the Best of Ward Nursing Resources. London: HMSO.

Barriball K, While A (1996) Participation in continuing professional education in nursing: findings of an interview study. Journal of Advanced Nursing 23: 999–1007.

Barriball K, While A, Norman I (1992) Continuing professional education for qualified nurses: a review of the literature. Journal of Advanced Nursing 21: 1129–40.

Bircumshaw D (1990) The utilisation of research findings in clinical practice. Journal of Advanced Nursing 15: 1272–80.

Black N (1998) Clinical governance: fine words or action? British Medical Journal 316: 297–8.

Brown S, Grimes D (1995) A meta-analysis of nurse practitioners and nurse midwives in primary care. Nursing Research 44: 332–9.

Camiah S (1997) Utilization of nursing research in practice and application strategies to raise research awareness amongst nurse practitioners: a model for success. Journal of Advanced Nursing 26: 1193–202.

Capel S (1998) Nurses' access to library and information services. Nursing Standard 12(25): 45–7.

Carper B (1978) Fundamental patterns of knowing in nursing. Advances in Nursing Science 1: 13–23.

Corbett K (1998) The captive market in nurse education and the displacement of nursing knowledge. Journal of Advanced Nursing 28: 524–31.

Cullum N, DiCenso A, Ciliska D (1998) Evidence-based practice. Nursing Management 5: 32–5.

Davis D, Thomson M, Oxman A, Haynes R (1995) Changing physician performance: A systematic review of the effect of continuing medical education strategies. Journal of the American Medical Association 274: 700–5.

Department of Health (1989) Working for Patients: Education and Training – Working Paper 10. London: DoH.

Department of Health (1993) Vision for the Future: The Nursing, Midwifery and Health Visiting Contribution to Health and Health Care. London: DoH.

Department of Health (1998a) The New NHS – Working Together: Securing a Quality Workforce for the NHS. London: DoH.

Department of Health (1998b) Our Healthier Nation: A Government Green Paper. London: HMSO.

Department of Health (1999) Making a Difference: Strengthening the Nursing, Midwifery and Health Visiting Contribution to Health and Healthcare. London: DoH.

Dunn V, Crichton N, Roe B, Seers K, Williams K (1997) Using research for practice: a UK experience of the BARRIERS Scale. Journal of Advanced Nursing 26: 1203–10.

Elliott P, Pickering S (1997) The purpose of PREP. Nursing Management 4: 12–13.

English National Board (1990) Framework for Continuing Professional Education for Nurses, Midwives and Health Visitors, Guide to Implementation. London: ENB.

Farmer J, Richardson A (1997) Information for trained nurses in remote areas: do electronically networked systems provide the answer? Health Libraries Review 14: 97–103.

Fennessey G (1998) Access route. Nursing Standard 12(18): 26–7.

Fitzpatrick J, While A, Roberts J (1994) The measurement of nurse performance and its differentiation by course of preparation. Journal of Advanced Nursing 20: 761–8.

Flemming K, Cullum N (1997) Doing the right thing. Nursing Standard 12(7): 28–30.

Furze G, Pearcey P (1999) Continuing education in nursing: a review of the literature. Journal of Advanced Nursing 29: 355–63.

Godbolt S, Williamson J, Wilson A (1997) From vision to reality – Managing change in the provision of library and information service to nurses, midwives, health visitors and PAMs: a case study of the North Thames experience with the Inner London Consortium. Health Libraries Review 14: 73–95.

Griffiths P (1996) Clinical outcomes for nurse led inpatient care. Nursing Times 92(9): 40–3.

Hogston R (1995) Nurses' perceptions of the impact of continuing professional education on the quality of nursing care. Journal of Advanced Nursing 22: 586–93.

Houghton G (1997) From audit to effectiveness: an historical evaluation of the changing role of Medical Audit Advisory Groups. Journal of Evaluation in Clinical Practice 3: 245–53.

Humphreys J (1996) Education commissioning by consortia: some theoretical and practical issues relating to qualitative aspects of British nurse education. Journal of Advanced Nursing 24: 1288–99.

Hunt J (1981) Indicators for nursing practice. Journal of Advanced Nursing 16: 89–114.

Ibbotson T, Grimshaw J, Grant A (1998) Evaluation of a programme of workshops for promoting the teaching of critical appraisal skills. Medical Education 32: 486–91.

Jordan S, Hughes D (1998) Using bioscience knowledge in nursing: actions, interactions and reactions. Journal of Advanced Nursing 27: 1060–18.

Kenny N (1997) Does good science make good medicine? Incorporating evidence into practice is complicated by the fact that clinical practice is as much art as science. Canadian Medical Association Journal 157(1): 33–6.

Kitson A (1997) Using evidence to demonstrate the value of nursing. Nursing Standard

11(28): 34–9.

McClarey M (1998) Implementing clinical effectiveness. Nursing Management 5(3): 16–19.

Maynard A (1988) The inefficiency and inequality of health care systems in Western Europe. In: Loney M, Boswell D, Clark J, eds. Social Policy and Social Welfare. Milton Keynes: Open University Press.

Moores Y, Jarrold K (1994) Nursing, Midwifery and Health Visiting Education – A Statement of Strategic Intent. London: Department of Health.

NHS Centre for Reviews and Dissemination (1999) Effective Health Care: Getting Evidence into Practice, Vol 5, number 1. York: University of York.

NHS Executive (1996) Clinical Guidelines: Using Clinical Guidelines to Improve Patient Care within the NHS. Leeds: NHS Executive.

NHS Executive (1998a) Effectiveness and cost effectiveness of teaching critical appraisal skills to clinicians, patients/users, purchasers and providers to promote uptake of research findings: [http://www.doh.gov/ntrd/rd/implem/priority/first/12.htm].

NHS Executive (1998b) Investigating educational strategies for continuing professional development to promote the implementation of research findings: [http://www.doh.gov.uk/ntrd/rd/implem/priority/first/11.htm].

Nolan M, Owens R, Nolan J (1995) Continuing professional education: identifying the characteristics of an effective system. Journal of Advanced Nursing 21: 551–60.

Oxman A, Thomson M, Davis D, Haynes R (1995) No magic bullets: a systematic review of 102 trials of interventions to improve professional practice. Canadian Medical Association Journal 153: 1423–31.

Pearcey P (1995) Achieving research-based nursing practice. Journal of Advanced Nursing 22: 33–9.

Regan JA (1998) Will current clinical effectiveness initiatives encourage and facilitate practitioners to use evidence-based practice for the benefit of their clients? Journal of Clinical Nursing 7: 244–50.

Sackett D, Rosenberg W (1995) Evidence-based Medicine and Guidelines in Clinical Effectiveness. From guidelines to cost effective practice. Manchester: Health Services Management Unit, University of Manchester.

Scally G, Donaldson L (1998) Looking forward: Clinical governance and the drive for quality improvement in the new NHS in England. British Medical Journal 317: 61–5.

Scheller M (1993) A qualitative analysis of factors in the work environment that influence nurses' use of knowledge gained from CE programmes. Journal of Continuing Education in Nursing 24: 114–22.

Smith J (1998) Exploring evidence-based practice: International conference organized by the University of Southampton School of Nursing and Midwifery at the Chilworth manor Conference Centre, Southampton, England, 12–14 September 1997 (Conference report). Journal of Advanced Nursing 27: 227–9.

Swage T (1998) Clinical care takes centre stage. Nursing Times 94(14): 40–1.

United Kingdom Central Council (1990) The Report of the Post-Registration Education and Practice Project. London: UKCC.

United Kingdom Central Council (1992a) The Code of Professional Practice. London: UKCC.

United Kingdom Central Council (1992b) The Scope of Professional Practice. London: UKCC.

United Kingdom Central Council (1994) The Future of Professional Practice: The Council's Standards for Education and Practice Following Registration. London: UKCC.

Waddell D (1991) The effects of continuing education on nursing practice: a meta-analysis. Journal of Continuing Education in Nursing 22: 113–18.

Walshe K, Ford P (1995) Nursing Rituals – Research and Rational Actions. Oxford: Butterworth-Heinemann.

Walshe K, Ham C (1997) Who's acting on the evidence? Health Service Journal 107: 22–5.

Webb C, Mackenzie J (1993) Where are we now? Research mindedness in the 1990's. Journal of Clinical Nursing 2: 129–33.

Wildman S, Weale A, Rodney C, Pritchard J (1999) The impact of higher education for post registration nurses on their subsequent clinical practice: an exploration of student's views. Journal of Advanced Nursing 29(1): 246–53.

Chapter 5
The partnership agenda

Jane Dawson

In earlier chapters we considered how changes to the management and organisational structures of the NHS, in addition to increasing emphasis on professional accountability for practice, have all been aimed at improving not only how well health care was delivered, but also the effectiveness of the clinical care itself. However, alongside these there has been a more subtle, but no less vital, policy shift, which recognises that the complexities of health care cannot always be met by the provision of health services in isolation.

Partnership

Government policy and legislation from 1995 onwards has placed great emphasis on the concept of partnership. This is being applied to partnerships between different organisational structures within the NHS itself, but also to partnerships between the NHS and other agencies. Just what does this mean and how will it work in practice? More importantly, from the point of view of this book, how does it affect or influence the concept of clinical effectiveness and clinical governance in clinical practice? Let us first look at partnerships between the NHS and other agencies

Partnerships with other agencies

For some patients, their experience of care is a visit to their GP, a course of treatment and then recovery. For others, care and treatment are ongoing, because their condition is long term or chronic. Nevertheless, it is dealt with largely by the GP, with input perhaps from the practice nurse or community nurse. Some require referral to specialist facilities, either for inpatient treatment or outpatient care. Whatever the progress of the episode, care and treatment are entirely within the NHS.

For many people, however, particularly chronically sick individuals, children, and elderly or vulnerable people, the ongoing care and services required are outside the remit of the NHS. This might include help with domestic work, special aids and adaptations to the home, day care, special housing or respite services for carers. Clearly, if the experience of patients and their carers is to be one of good quality and effective services, a great deal of cooperation and collaboration are required between a large number of different agencies and disciplines.

In addition, the nature of health care has changed, with early discharge, day surgery, etc. The average inpatient stay for patients admitted to acute services fell from 11.3 days in 1970 to 8.6 in 1980 and 6.1 days in 1990 – exclusive of day cases (NHS E, 1996a). Thus, there is a growing need for timely and efficient transfer across the primary/secondary interface and between NHS and other agencies, while these changes themselves mean that there is less time in which to communicate the information.

Consider the case of an elderly woman who has been in hospital for a fractured neck of femur.

Challenge: Write down all the different disciplines that would be involved in her care while in hospital. Now add all those that may be needed when she is discharged.

Now think of a child born with severe cerebral palsy. His parents already have two other children and his father has diabetes. The child is unable to walk, but has some speech and a normal intelligence.

Challenge: What agencies are likely to be involved in the child's care and that of the family by the time he is aged 10 years?

In 1998, the Department of Health issued a discussion document *Partnership in Action (New Opportunities for Joint Working between Health and Social Services)* (Department of Health, 1998a). This set out in detail how organisational and budgetary arrangements could be managed so as to provide coordinated services. The intention was to put paid to problems encountered all too frequently concerning geographical and budgetary boundaries. Joint working was advocated at three levels:

1. Planning
2. Commissioning services
3. Providing services.

The document (Department of Health, 1998a) states that the proposals must also:

- improve the actual services that users and carers receive;
- ensure that wasteful duplication and gaps in services are avoided;
- ensure that public funds are used more efficiently and effectively.

What has this to do with clinical governance and clinical effectiveness? Think back to the definitions of clinical governance and clinical effectiveness discussed in Chapter 1. Dunning and Ayres' (1998) definition of clinical governance was:

> Clinical Governance places expectations and responsibilities on individuals and organisations to put in place systems to ensure the delivery of high quality health care to patients.

The NHS Executive Letter (1995) defined clinical effectiveness as:

> The extent to which specific clinical interventions, when deployed in the field for a particular patient or population, do what they are intended to do – i.e. maintain and improve health and secure the greatest possible gain from available resources.

Take our examples of an elderly patient and a physically disabled child. Their care needs can be clinically effective and efficiently met and 'wasteful duplication and gaps in services avoided' (Department of Health, 1998b) only if the various agencies who supply the required services ensure that plans are coordinated and communicated, so that everyone can be sure that they are doing the right thing right (Kitson, 1998).

What does all this mean for nurses, midwives, GPs and practice nurses? For a start, it means such staff will have to be much more prepared to share information and discuss plans concerning patient care with other disciplines. Patients and their carers must be seen as the hub of a 'care wheel', with the agencies involved acting as the spokes that provide support, each spoke having its unique part to play. If one spoke gives way, the wheel ceases to function. In theory, the huge advances in information technology, such as links with hospital pathology laboratories, patient-held electronic medical summaries, new computer systems in general practice, electronic transfer of records, email and mobile phones should make this easier, rather than relying as in the past on letters or telephone. In practice, this will work only if all those involved make use of such systems to pass on important information

---

Example

A Community Hospital Unit for Adults with Learning Disabilities was due for upgrading. Although clients and their families appeared happy with the work of the unit, it was decided to take the opportunity to review the scope of the care provided and to make sure that it met the needs of clients, carers and the local community. A survey showed that families and carers were keen to be involved in the upgrade project and wanted clients to be included as well.

Actions
- A meeting was held for families at which plans for the upgrade were discussed, and their views sought, on the building itself, its facilities and the way the unit would operate in future.
- Clients at the unit were shown a model of the new building and key workers looked for opportunities to gain and record their views on the building and on the things that they would like to see incorporated. Clients were encouraged to make a statement about what they liked abut the unit and what they would like to change.
- A meeting was held for Social Services, the local education authority, the relevant voluntary associations (e.g. **MIND**), the

Community Health Council (CHC), the nursing department at the university, teachers from a local feeder school and a number of community nurses and local GPs. Views on the service currently offered and what changes were needed were sought by means of a questionnaire.

Findings
• Families expressed the need for more training on dealing with people with learning disabilities as they approached adulthood. Teachers also felt that this would be helpful.
• Some families also saw a need for some form of outreach service for teenagers who would be attending the unit later on.

Many of the statutory and voluntary agencies supported this view.

• Facilities for clients who became ill were rather patchy. Nursing staff at the unit often found themselves caring for clients without being clear what the problem was or how to deal with it.
• Both families and clients wanted to have a say in the day-to-day running of the unit.
• Clients also wanted more opportunities for physical activity, such as dancing, swimming and sports.

Changes
• A Management Committee was formed, with carer, client, nursing staff and other agency representatives. Clients also had their own House Committee.
• A new timetable was drawn up, which included sessions for dancing and trips to the local swimming pool. A Sports Club was formed.
• Joint training programmes were instigated for staff, families and other interested individuals.
• A Home Visiting scheme was established whereby senior staff visited potential clients.
• The local health centre agreed to provide advice and support to staff when clients became ill.

Results a year later

- Clients now elect their own Chairperson of the House Committee, who is helped by his or her key worker to carry out the role.
- The Management Committee makes decisions on the running of the centre, staff appointments and a number of other management functions, as well as fund-raising and other events. The House Committee Chairperson is a member of the Management Committee.
- The university nursing department is developing the curriculum for an NVQ, which will be offered to all those undertaking the unit's training programme, including families.
- The Sports Team is aiming to compete in a number of national events for athletes with learning disabilities.
- All potential clients are visited at home or school by a member of staff.
- The health centre was unable to undertake its support role, but a named member of the unit's staff is now responsible for liaising with the relevant GP and community nurses.

In this situation, a number of agencies had a relevant contribution to make about the future running of the unit, as well as families and clients. Cooperation and sharing of information have improved services to clients and their families.

The Caldicott Committee

There is another aspect of information sharing that must be borne in mind, however. A review was commissioned in 1997 by the Chief Medical Officer of England, to look at the way patient information is used in the NHS and how the need to ensure confidentiality is maintained. The Review Committee examined patient information flows and made 16 recommendations (NHS E, 1997) to support good practice principles.

How does the principle of clinical governance apply here? The clinical effectiveness framework considered in Chapter 1 (NHS Executive Letter, 1995) was inform, change and monitor. Although this cannot be applied directly to the joint working arrangements set out in the partnership document, there are similarities in the monitoring, reviewing and holding to account that this specifies. Another point is that the agencies involved in complex situations may be statutory (Social Services, the NHS) or voluntary (Age Concern, MIND). All must learn to work together, but voluntary agencies are not subject to the same statutory authority, inspection and reporting as Social Services and the NHS. How such very different organisations, with their spectrum of philosophies, cultures and value systems, are to come together in this way is outside the scope of this book. However, the issue of monitoring is one that we need to consider.

The monitoring of both the NHS and Social Services

How can the care received by the elderly woman or by the child and his family be evaluated? How will it be decided whether the services provided have been good value for money, whether the options offered were the most effective available, and whether the care and services given have improved health outcomes and lifestyle? More importantly, who will make the judgement? The partnership document (Department of Health, 1998b) refers to 'Performance Frameworks' for the NHS and Social Services Authorities, which was published by the NHS Executive in 1998 (Department of Health, 1998b; NHS E, 1998). This specifies how services are to be measured in future, so health authorities, NHS trusts, Social Services departments and voluntary organisations will need to have systems and processes in place to make sure that the quality and effectiveness of their services are continuously assessed and that lessons are learned. In addition, however adequate such systems are in practice, both the partnership document and the performance frameworks stress the importance of involving patients and families in evaluation and audit of the services that they receive.

Challenge: What mechanisms could be used to gain the views of the elderly woman on the care she received both while in hospital and after discharge?

In answer to this, you probably came up with the methods listed below:

- satisfaction questionnaires;
- clinical audit of care in hospital;
- periodic review to see whether home care is being delivered as planned;
- reassessment of need to ensure that services provided are still relevant;
- interview by independent researcher.

Some of these methods are easier to use than others. Patient satisfaction questionnaires are probably the most popular, but it is all too easy to design these so that they contain only questions that professionals think are relevant and, in any case, it is very difficult to gain meaningful views from patients about their clinical care in this way. Clinical audit is usually an entirely professional activity and the idea of including patients could be seen as inappropriate and, indeed, threatening. Periodic review and reassessment should be part of good practice but, if lessons are to be learned about services overall, someone needs to be drawing such material together. Independent research can be very valuable, but it goes without saying that it is costly and requires considerable effort to set up.

How can patients be drawn into the monitoring and evaluative process? One way is to try to identify what the most important issues for patients in a particular situation are, and then to incorporate these into the tools employed by professionals to audit their own work. This can be done by independent interview, using patient/client groups drawn together for this purpose, consulting patient and consumer organisations, establishing anonymous suggestion schemes and similar initiatives. Whatever the method employed, what is no longer an option is for staff to make no effort to gain patient views in the evaluation of care, and not to take these into account when plans for the future are developed.

Partnership within the NHS

Patient partnership

When the NHS was first established, all health-care professionals were looked on with some awe. Patients who visited the doctor or nurse, or who were admitted to hospital, would not have thought of questioning those providing care about what they were doing or why. Medical control of decision-making has been reported as still being the predominant model (Caress 1997; Coulter, 1997). In addition, the treatment delivered by one professional, e.g. the doctor, was seen as separate from the care given by the nurse or the physiotherapist. Professionals did not automatically discuss patients with each other, share clinical records or coordinate the advice that they were giving to the patient. During the 1990s, attitudes and philosophy began to change fundamentally. This was very much in line with a move to increased consumer awareness and rights, and a growing recognition that sometimes healthcare professionals made mistakes (Hickey, 1986).

The idea of patient partnership became prominent with the publication of *Working for Patients* (Department of Health, 1989), in which it was proposed that consumer views should be taken into account in the planning and delivery of services. The introduction of the Patient's Charter in 1991 (Department of Health, 1991) took that a stage further, because it set out the rights to health services and the standard of such services that every member of the public could expect to receive. It was thus a clear recognition that patients had views on health services, both as individual recipients of care and as members of the wider community at local and national levels.

In the main, the rights set out in the Patients' Charter are fairly broad brush, e.g. the right to be registered with a GP, and the right to be prescribed appropriate medicines and drugs. Standards too are similarly basic, such as the expectation that community nurses will consult patients about a convenient time for their visit, or that parents can expect their child to be admitted to a paediatric ward. Nevertheless, the Patient's Charter signalled a departure from previous attitudes towards patients, in that it made explicit the fact that the role of patients within health services was in future to be as an active participant, rather than a passive recipient.

Patient participation was a central plank of Government policy in the Priorities and Planning Guidelines document for 1996–97 (NHS Executive Letter, 1995). These Guidelines, stated in future NHS organisations, must:

> Give greater voice and influence to users of NHS services and their carers in their own care, the development and definition of standards set for NHS services locally and the development of NHS policy both locally and nationally.

The guidelines went on to set out what health authorities and service providers were expected to do to meet this. These included such things as planning to communicate and consult local people and groups on development of local services, and encouraging the production of information to patients to enable them to make choices about treatment options.

This was followed in 1996 by the publication, by the NHS Executive, of *Patient Partnership: Building a Collaborative Strategy* (NHS E, 1996a). This laid out in detail what was being done to implement the priority statement in the Priorities and Planning Guidelines (NHS Management Executive, 1995). It listed the reasons behind this priority:

- If services are developed on the basis of need identified by users, they are more likely to be appropriate and effective.
- Patients, carers and the public expect more say in the development of the NHS, what is provided and to what standard.
- Patients want more information about their own care and to have more choice in the treatment options open to them. This supports the concept of informed consent.
- There is evidence that patient outcomes and satisfaction are improved if they are more involved in their own care.
- Evaluation of clinical effectiveness and health outcomes must include patient perspectives on benefit.

It is now an expectation of Central Government that primary care groups will involve NHS users and the public. Patients will be represented on the National Institute for Clinical Excellence and on the Commission for Health Improvement. Public involvement in planning and development of local health services will be part of the Health Improvement Programmes agenda.

Example

A local, much-loved hospital was due for closure. Its buildings were out of date and in need of repair. The focal point of residential areas had shifted over time, so that the hospital was difficult for many young families to get to. The Local Health Authority wanted to replace it with new purpose-built premises. The question was exactly what purpose would the new facility serve? What did the local community really want?

Action

The Health Authority decided to hold a series of half-day events, to which a wide cross-section of the public would be invited. Letters were sent to local schools and play groups, GPs, dentists, pharmacists, voluntary organisations such as Age Concern and youth groups, the CHC, the Acute and Community NHS Trusts, Social Services and the education authority, local religious groups and the business community, as well as the 'Save our Hospital' group. The local press and radio publicised the events, sent a representative and published a major feature article on each one. The public was invited to write or phone in with their comments.

The events were held in the Art Centre, refreshments were provided and there was a crèche for those with children, to encourage participation by younger families. The events were carefully structured, the first being to identify what people liked about the hospital, what they did not like and what they felt was missing. At the next session, the Health Authority talked through what they saw as priorities for services in future, and people were asked to rank the order of importance that they attached to each. At later sessions, the results of this exercise were fed back, a list of 'Top Choices' drawn up and subgroups discussed these and reported back to the main arena. At the final session, the health authority put forward its plans in the light of all the discussion.

Result

The closure went ahead, but most of the local community felt that they had been properly consulted on what should take its place. The services ultimately provided were different in several ways to those that the Health Authority had planned and arrangements were made for more outreach facilities in a number of health centres, community centres and business premises. A number of the participants formed the now flourishing 'Bloomington-on-Sea Health Care Support Group'.

The health authority could have just sought the views of the Acute and Community NHS Trust managers and local GPs. However, every member of the population in that area was a potential user of health services. What we must ask ourselves is just what do we mean by patients and what is participation? Iskander (1997) points out that a number of different words are used interchangeably in such discussions: service user, consumer, client, patient. All have subtly different connotations, but there is no shared understanding of their use. Similarly, empowerment, participation, collaboration, consultation and involvement are all employed to describe an active, rather than a passive, role. Cahill (1998) agrees, citing patient collaboration, patient involvement and patient partnership as terms used synonymously and comes to the conclusion that:

> There is no clear consensus on what patient participation means or how far it should be extended.

The King's Fund (Farrell and Gilbert, 1996) suggest a hierarchy of active roles. Involvement loosely describes any stage at which users are involved, at an individual or local level, in decision-making. Consultation describes attempts to seek users' views (hopefully at an early stage in planning). Participation is the highest level of activity, describing a much more dynamic approach in which various organisations and groups come together to reach decisions jointly. In the case of individuals, participation would mean patients having an equal say in decision-making about all aspects of care and treatment.

In an extensive review of the literature related to patient participation, Cahill (1998) argues that the *Working for Patients* document (Department of Health, 1989) was given added support by reforms in nursing practice, such as the nursing process, nursing models, primary nursing and a more patient-centred focus.

Before making the assumption that all patients wish to participate as much as possible in all circumstances, we need to be sure that this is in fact the case. Patients frequently remain passive recipients of care, because that has been the pattern in the past and, it is fair to say, because the professions themselves (Iskander, 1997; Cahill, 1998) have often discouraged them. Some studies have found that certain factors influence the role that patients choose to play with regard to participation. Brooking (1986) found that there was greater participation on the part of patients of higher social class, those who were younger and those who knew more about their condition. In a study of patients with renal disease, Caress (1997) demonstrated that, although the most popular single role was collaborative, most patients preferred a passive role. In particular, more elderly people showed greater deference to health professionals and being 'too ill' was also seen as a reason to minimise participation. This study, along with others (Coulter, 1997), did show, however, that patients wanted information, even if they played a passive role in decision-making. What this means in practice is that nurses must not coerce patients into active participation in making decisions about their care, but offer information, encouraging and supporting patients in their choice of role.

Challenge: What information is made available to patients in your clinical area? What form does this take? List all the ways in which there is patient participation in clinical decision-making. What role do they take – user, consumer, etc. – and what is the level of their commitment – involved, consulted, etc.? How is their role negotiated?

Does all this matter and how does it fit in to clinical effectiveness?

Well, first, if evaluation of the clinical effectiveness of care is to have any real meaning, it must include the perception of those who receive that care. That old joke 'the operation was a success but the patient died' comes to mind. Are we sure at the outset of treatment whether the patient knows what the anticipated outcome is and whether it is what he or she really wants? If not, how can we measure whether the treatment was effective or not? Who is to judge? Second, if we are going to start discussing with colleagues how we can encourage users to participate in decisions about their care, we need to ensure that we are all talking about the same thing and have a shared understanding of the concepts that we are trying to convey and the words that we employ to describe them.

It is at this point that we have to consider the way in which care is organised and delivered. If Mrs Smith was asked how good her care was, she would make the judgement on all the care provided, not just that in hospital, or what happened when she got home. Perhaps she feels that she had very good care, but she had to wait for 2 hours while her drugs to take home were prepared. She was discharged on a Friday, but the 'Meals on Wheels' did not start until the following Wednesday, although they were very nice when they did come. The hospital transport was late arriving to take her to the outpatients appointment and, as she was late, she had to wait 2 hours to be seen, but the driver was helpful and the nurse gave her a cup of tea. Her leg healed well and she is walking again. Has the care she received been clinically effective or not?

Such a scenario is extremely simplistic, but it does serve to make the point that the quality and effectiveness of care are increasingly dependent, not just on individuals, but on teamwork.

Partnership between disciplines: multidisciplinary teams

Much of the literature on multidisciplinary teams is based on research in a primary care setting (Robison and Wiles, 1994; West and Slater, 1996). Perhaps this is caused by the organisational system in which care is delivered. A general practice, which is geographically located in a surgery or health centre, has a number of different disciplines either working under one roof, such as the doctors, practice nurses, receptionists and practice manager, or identified with it, such as 'attached' community nurses, health visitors, psychiatric nurses and physiotherapists. There is a clearly identified client/patient group – all those registered with that practice – who remain for months, years, maybe a lifetime. In a hospital or community trust setting, although all these disciplines work within them, they are physically distributed around the building or buildings. Various disciplines come together at intervals to consider a specific client group (e.g. patients on an orthopaedic ward) or individuals (e.g. a psychiatric patient). The rest of the time, individual health professionals may be involved with a quite different client group, even a different hospital. Medical staff are the predominant discipline (Rodgers, 1994) and organisation is largely departmental and hierarchical.

Why teams don't work

Drawing on research into multidisciplinary teams (Brooking, 1986; Rodgers, 1994; West and Slater, 1996), we can identify a number of factors that prevent them developing and working together.

Poor communication
This can result from lack of time to arrange meetings or send information.

Medical domination
Many doctors feel, with some justification, that because they are ultimately legally responsible for the patients' care, they need to retain overall control.

Power differentials

Medical staff are generally perceived as having more power than nurses and other health professionals. Other disciplines, such as social workers or community nurses visiting a ward or GP practice may feel they have little or no power or status within that environment.

Varied management of team members

Community nurses, health visitors and other professionals 'attached' to primary health care report through their own management structure, outside the GP practice. The same is usually true of nurses, physiotherapists and others in the acute and community care sectors, even where there is a shared client group or service, such as psychiatric outpatients or a paediatric ward.

Low management commitment

Given the different management systems, all managers must be equally committed to 'their' staff working in a team model if such an approach is to work.

Different location of team members

Although nurses are located and work on specific wards or within specific service areas, physiotherapists, medical staff and others are usually peripatetic, with their own department and office.

Divergent values, philosophies and training

The specific body of knowledge and skill sets that go to make up a professional identity itself creates different cultures, ideologies and perspectives. Thus, doctors are trained to a predominantly medical model which emphasises biological and physiological systems, nurses increasingly adopt and are trained in a more holistic model of care, whereas the prime concerns of social workers are the social and emotional needs of an individual.

Different priorities

Given this variation in outlook, even health-care professionals working with the same patient or client group are likely to have different priorities and goals, which may cause conflict.

What is a team?

If, however, we look at what constitutes a team, there is no overriding reason why multidisciplinary teams should not operate in acute and community settings. West and Slater (1996) suggest that groups of workers should have certain characteristics to be identified as a team:

- collective responsibility for shared aims and objectives;
- systems and opportunities to interact with each other;
- well-defined and differentiated roles of individuals;
- a clear identity as a work team.

Challenge: What disciplines have input to the clinical area in which you work? How many of the characteristics of teams do you feel apply to them?

It would seem that the various disciplines that provide care to inpatients on a ward, clients in a group home or outpatients attending a diabetes clinic have, or should have, the first three characteristics. What they lack is the last, a clear identity as a work team. In a study of primary health care teams, Robison and Wiles (1994) described three levels of team development, which they describe as individualistic, GP-led and democratic. Although all practices recognised the need in principle to work as a team, active moves to achieve this varied. Below is a fictional example of how a team can work together to improve patient care and make it more clinically and cost-effective.

Example

The staff in an ear, nose and throat clinic were concerned that they were not offering patients referred with hearing loss the best possible service. An audit and service review found the following problems:

- Waiting times were 17–26 weeks between first and follow-up appointments.
- A 15% non-attendance rate.
- Clinics were overbooked.
- Forty per cent of tests were considered unnecessary and 20%

were repeated without clear purpose at the second appointment. Test results were frequently lost. The department pathology budget was badly overspent.

- Nurses spent 30% of their time looking for notes and test results.
- Information provided to patients, GPs and other staff and agencies was conflicting, confused and often late in arriving.

Action

A team was formed, which included every member of staff who worked in the clinic, as well as the service manager. This covered medical staff, nurses, audiologists, medical records staff, appointment clerks and a GP. A project plan was drawn up, and the team divided into subgroups:

- Group 1 mapped the patient pathway from referral to treatment.
- Group 2 reviewed the content and dissemination of information.
- Group 3 searched the literature for evidence of the usefulness of the tests being administered and for any guidelines on best practice.
- Group 4 conducted a patient survey and held a patient focus group.

Findings

It became apparent that some work within the clinic was duplicated, although it was unclear who was responsible for carrying out other tasks. There was no evidence to support the administration of about half the tests routinely administered in the clinic, which had often required a repeat appointment. The current system of notifying GPs of the planned follow-up caused unnecessary delay. Patients found the delays upsetting and wanted the opportunity to discuss the options for treatment more fully.

Changes

- Guidelines were drawn up for future clinical practice and on the type and frequency of clinical tests.
- A senior nurse was identified to interview patients at the end of their first appointment to answer questions and explain treatment choices.

- Wherever possible, arrangements were made to fax or email letters through to GPs, with copies to other relevant agencies or individuals, such as teachers or Social Services.
- New information leaflets were drawn up for patients, which were to be sent out with the first appointment.
- Test results were to be returned to the clinic via the hospital-wide computer system.
- A streamlined system for storage and retrieval of records was designed.
- All staff roles and responsibilities were clarified.

Results
- Non-attendance dropped to 5%.
- Nurses no longer spent time obtaining notes.
- Care was given and tests conducted in accordance with the guidelines in 95% of cases. Only 3% of test results were mislaid.
- GPs were notified of findings and treatment plans within 2 days of the first appointment.
- Clinics were no longer overbooked because unnecessary visits were eliminated.
- A patient survey found greatly increased levels of satisfaction with the service.

Only by working together could the clinic staff ensure that their care was efficient, timely and effective, and that patients were satisfied with the outcomes of care. A variety of methods was used to collect data on what was happening and what should happen. Changes were then instituted and the results reviewed. Although this case study is fictional, it is not that dissimilar from many real-life situations.

In primary care it is possible, indeed likely, that team working will develop within primary care groups as they grow in stature and influence. Certainly, all the factors identified earlier as necessary for building teams should be present. In fact, it is difficult to see how a primary care group could operate effectively unless such things were in place, both between and within the various general practices.

Conclusion

All this paints a rather confusing and somewhat challenging picture. Are we ready to have old beliefs, attitudes and values threatened? How will we cope with patients who choose not to take the treatment option that we consider best for them? Will we cling to familiar and traditional professional hierarchies? We should remember that things are already changing rapidly. There is an increasing tendency for training, at both the basic or undergraduate level and more advanced professional development to be delivered jointly to more than one discipline. Thus, student nurses and medical students may have joint lectures on patient attitudes, or physiotherapists and nurses attend the same course on clinical audit. Management structures are nowadays more likely to be organised around patient groups – diabetes services or paediatric home care – although this clearly cuts across traditional hierarchies. Information technology is reshaping the way that patient information is recorded and processed. Health Authorities, Trusts and Social Services departments have been given specific targets and criteria by which to monitor their performance, so 'turf wars' between agencies will become counterproductive. Most important of all is the emerging role of patients and the general public, with primary care at the hub. If patients become the focal point of service organisation and service delivery, playing an active role in decision-making about their own care and the development of services in and for their community, this has the potential to be the biggest force for change in the 50 years of the NHS's existence. Nurses must be ready to meet this change and recognise the opportunity that it presents to develop truly effective nursing practice.

References

Brooking J (1986) A survey of current practice and opinions concerning patient and family participation in hospital care. In: Wilson-Barnett J, Robinson S, eds. Directions in Nursing Research. Harrow: Scutari Press.

Cahill J (1998) Patient participation – a review of the literature. Journal of Clinical Nursing 7: 119–28.

Caress A (1997) Patient roles in decision making. Nursing Times 93(31): 45–8.

Coulter A (1997) Partnerships with patients: the pros and cons of shared clinical decision-making. Journal of Health Services Research and Policy 2: 112–21.

Department of Health (1989) Working for Patients: The Health Service Caring for the 1990s. London: HMSO.

Department of Health (1991) The Patient's Charter. London: HMSO.

Department of Health (1998a) National Service Frameworks. London Health Service Circular: HSC 1998/074.

Department of Health (1998b) Partnership in Action (New Opportunities for Joint Working between Health and Social Services). Leeds: DoH.

Dunning M, Ayers P (1998) What is clinical governance? – a workable definition. Healthcare Quality 4(3): 16–18.

Farrell C, Gilbert H (1996) Healthcare Partnerships. London: King's Fund.

Hickey T (1986) Health behaviour and self care in later life. In: Dean K, Hickey T, Holstein B, eds. Self Care and Health in Old Age. London: Croom Helm.

Iskander R (1997) User involvement: from principles to practice. Health Visitor 70: 455–7.

Kitson A (1998) The Government White Papers: A view from nursing. Healthcare Quality 4(1): 5–9.

NHS E (1996a) Patient Partnership: Building a Collaborative Strategy. Leeds: NHS Executive.

NHS E (1996b) Patient Partnership: Building a Collaborative Strategy. Leeds: NHS Executive.

NHS E (1997) The Caldicott Committee Report on the review of patient-identifiable information. Leeds: NHS Executive.

NHS E (1998) The New NHS: Modern and Dependable: A National Framework for Assessing Performance. Leeds: Department of Health.

NHS Executive Letter (1995) Improving the Effectiveness of Clinical Services. EL (95) 105. London: NHS Executive.

NHS Management Executive (1995) Priorities and Planning Guidance for the NHS: 1996/97. EL (95) 68. London: NHS Executive.

Robison J, Wiles R (1994) Teamwork in Primary Care: Do Patients Benefit? Institute for Health Policy Research, University of Southampton.

Rodgers J (1994) Collaboration among health professionals. Nursing Standard 9(6): 25–6.

West M, Slater J (1996) Teamwork in Primary Health Care: A Review of its Effectiveness. London: Health Education Authority.

Chapter 6
Resources available – or where do I start?

JANE DAWSON

By the time you have got this far in the book you will, hopefully, have some understanding of how the principle of clinical effectiveness came about and what it means for you and your clinical practice, for nurse education and for professional development. You will also have begun to understand how the evidence on which effective practice is based is found, evaluated and synthesised, and the way in which the organisation and delivery of health care may change. What this chapter considers is where do you go from here? How do you find the evidence on which to base your particular practice, or plan a programme of improvements in your clinical area?

You could begin by asking the Alice in Wonderland question: 'How do I know how to get there if I don't know where I'm going?' In other words, what is it you want to achieve? Does your clinical area have a particular problem with which you wish to deal? Are you less than satisfied with the outcomes of care for a specific client or patient group? Do you suspect that care could be better organised? As with research, the first stage is to define the question or problem that you wish to tackle clearly. Then you can start to look for appropriate resources to assist you.

Begin by considering what resources there are within your trust, GP practice or community service. Is there a clinical audit department or audit facilitator? Some of these have moved on and are now called clinical effectiveness departments, or they may be part of the quality assurance or quality improvement department. Whatever their title, seek them out, and go and discuss your ideas with them. These people have been specially trained to help you improve your practice and the service you deliver, but they can do this only if they know what help is required. There may already be an active clinical audit or Continuous Quality Improvement programme in your area. Find out about it and see how you can get involved. You will probably find that this department runs various training courses to help practitioners to learn and practise the skills necessary to introduce and maintain evidence-based practice. Quite often, such courses are geared to the needs of a multidisciplinary team working in a specific clinical area, so that all the health professionals involved can learn and work together.

Another avenue is through postgraduate training or in-service training. Again, find out what is available and, if there is a postgraduate clinical tutor, go and speak to him or her. Such courses may be open to a particular profession, e.g. nurses, midwives or physiotherapists, but others may be more multidisciplinary in nature. Sometimes the training on offer is focused around tackling a specific clinical issue, so you could practise your new skills with the support of the tutor and other students.

You could also find out if your trust or service has a research and development unit, or a link with such a unit, maybe with another trust or a local university. Again, the people here may be able to offer advice and expertise.

What are the mechanisms for discussing your thoughts and ideas with your immediate colleagues? Is there a journal club, or a current awareness noticeboard? Do you have ward, clinic or team meetings? Is there a special interest group that you could join? If not, why not start one yourself? Could you invite a respected senior colleague to come to a meeting to talk to the group about how to proceed in dealing with a problem or making some improvement?

Half an hour spent talking to those who are more experienced, or with the specialised skills, could save hours of aimless discussion and start to point you in the right direction.

As well as resources immediately to hand, find out what is available in the broader environment. What kind of services, advice and resources does the relevant library offer? Most will provide bibliography lists for a specific subject, such as rehabilitation, wound care, etc., either for particular professionals (e.g. nurses) or generic. Computer facilities in libraries have increased enormously in recent years, so that searching research databases, such as CINAHL or

MEDLINE, is now much easier. Libraries will also offer coaching sessions in how to go about searching, as this in itself is a skill that needs to be learned and practised. The library, particularly if it is attached to a medical or other professional school, will probably have an electronic link to other national clinical effectiveness sources of information.

How about the local branch of your professional organisation (e.g. Royal College of Nursing, Royal College of Midwives)? Many of these have active programmes to support, educate and advise members in improving their practice or services. If the local branch is not very active, contact the national headquarters to find out what is available.

Whatever help and support of this kind you are able to discover, you will inevitably need to utilise facilities at a national level. This is not as daunting as it may sound, because the whole point of these organisations is to act as a resource to practitioners, so they aim to be as user friendly as possible. You will find that you build up expertise on finding sources of information quite quickly. Once you get to this stage, you will need to start organising the sources that you locate very carefully, because otherwise you will waste a lot of time retracing your steps. If you have your own computer, make a habit of putting the Internet addresses of the most useful sites into the bookmark facility. If you rely on a shared computer, say in the library or at college, you could copy the addresses into a Word file and save this on your own floppy disk, and then you can refer to it the next time that you wish to conduct a search. For those with no computer access, a card index system will provide a means of recording such information, although it is more time-consuming to set up and maintain.

A range of available resources is set out below, listed alphabetically. It is not really practical to try and divide them up into publications, organisations, resource centres, etc., because electronic communication is developing so fast. Most organisations have a website and email nowadays or are rapidly setting them up, printed journals will probably have a website, and text of articles and other material can often be downloaded directly to another computer. Similarly, organisations that operate primarily through websites frequently publish reports or other documentation in hard copy. If your computer facilities are limited, don't despair! Addresses, telephone numbers or hard copy material are given where possible. The list below is not exhaustive and some sources may have changed Internet addresses or organisational arrangements since going to press. There are some organisations and institutions not listed which are more academic in nature, or which act in an advisory capacity to policy-makers. However, those given should provide a starting point for most practitioners with the help required for all practical purposes.

The list below has been compiled from a variety of sources. In particular the School of Health and Related Research (ScHARR), University of Sheffield is a very rich source of information and has been generous in sharing this.

Resources for finding information on clinical effectiveness

Aggressive Research Intelligence Facility (ARIF)

'Advancing the use of evidence on the effects of health care in the West Midlands', ARIF is a specialist unit based at the University of Birmingham. The first objective of ARIF is to provide timely access to, and advice on, existing reviews of research in response to particular problems.

Institute of Public and Environmental Health
University of Birmingham
27 Highfield Road
Edgbaston
Birmingham B15 3DP

http://www.hsrc.org.uk/links/arif/arifhome.htm

Bandolier

Produced monthly in Oxford for the NHS R&D Directorate. It contains points of evidence-based medicine by alphabetical index. Internet access currently free. Subscription required for the printed version.

http://www.jr2.ox.ac.uk:80/Bandolier

British Nursing Index (BNI)

BNI is a partnership of Bournemouth University Library and Information Service, Bournemouth University, Poole Hospital NHS Trust, Salisbury Health Care NHS Trust and the Royal College of Nursing. Subscription details from BNI Publications.

Bournemouth University Library and Information Service
Bournemouth University
Dorset House
Talbot Compus
Fern Barrow
Poole
Dorset BH12 5BB

http://www.bni.org.uk/cgi-bin/index.html.html

CASP: Critical Appraisal Skills Programme

This is a UK project that aims to help health service professionals develop skills to find, critically appraise and change practice in line with evidence of effectiveness, thus promoting the delivery of evidence-based health care. CASP runs half-day workshops, which introduce people to the ideas of evidence-based health care and to the related ideas of the Cochrane Collaboration. An interactive CD-ROM is being developed, giving opportunities for independent practice or learning.

Oxford Institute of Health Sciences
PO Box 777
Oxford OX3 7LF
Tel: 01865 226968

Centre for Evidence-based Child Health

The Centre is part of a national network of centres for evidence-based health care. The aim of the Centre is to increase the provision of effective and efficient child health care through an educational programme to paediatricians, nurses, general practitioners, health-care purchasers and others involved in child health. Introductory seminars, short courses, MSc modules, workshops for workplace groups and training secondments are available.

Institute for Child Health
Great Ormond Street
London WC1N 3JH

http://www.ich.bpmf.ac.uk/ebm/ebm.htm

Centre for Evidence-based Dentistry

The Centre is based at the Institute of Health Sciences in Oxford. The main objective is to promote the teaching, learning, practice and evaluation of evidence-based dentistry throughout the UK.

http://www.bhaoral.demon.co.uk/

Centre for Evidence-based Medicine

Established in Oxford as the first of several centres around the country. The aim of these centres is to promote evidence-based health care and provide support and resources to professionals and academics. Covers public health, primary care, hospital medicine, child health, neonatology, mental health, surgery, obstetrics and gynaecology. Mainly for the medical profession.

Nuffield Department of Clinical Medicine
Level 5
The Oxford Radcliffe NHS Trust
Headley Way
Headington
Oxford OX3 9DV
Tel: 01865 222 941

http://cebm.jr2.ox.ac.uk/

Centre for Evidence-based Mental Health

Provides resources to promote and support the teaching and practice of evidence-based mental health care: provides links to evidence-based mental health websites; teaching resources; details of the journal *Evidence-based Mental Health;* information on workshops and conferences; details of how to join or subscribe to the mailing list. Future plans include information on the Network for Clinical Effectiveness and Evidence-based Practice, including the Royal College of Psychiatrists' clinical practice guidelines and a glossary of evidence-based medical terminology relevant to mental health.

http://www.psychiatry.ox.ac.uk/cebmh/frames.html

Centre for Evidence-based Nursing

Works with nurses in practice, researchers, nurse educators and managers to identify evidence-based practice. Undertakes research and systematic reviews, promotes the uptake of evidence into practice through education and other strategies. Also researches factors that promote or impede implementation of evidence-based practice. Based at the University of York, this Centre is part of the national network of Centres for Evidence-Based Clinical Practice Health Care.

http://www.york.ac.uk/depts/hstd/centres/evidence/ev-intro.htm

Centre for Evidence-based Pharmacotherapy

This was set up in July 1995 within the Department of Pharmaceutical Sciences, University of Nottingham to undertake research in the methodology of medicines assessment, pharmacoepidemiology and pharmacoeconomics (MAPP). The Centre is part of the Cochrane Collaboration, with membership of the editorial team of the Menstrual Disorders Review Group and the Statistical Methods Working Group. Coordinates the Pharmaceuticals Field. The Centre also has close links with the Consumers Association.

http://www.nottingham.ac.uk/~paxjc/clinphar.htm

CHAIN: Contact Help Advice Information Network for Effective Healthcare

A reference database for clinical effectiveness and evidence-based health care activities in the North Thames Region and beyond.

http://www.nthames-health.tpmde.ac.uk/chain/chain.htm

CINAHL

The main database for all nursing and other healthcare professionals' research. Most university libraries will have access to this, but if you want to establish your own link you will have to register.

www.cinahl.com

Clinical Audit and Resources Group (CRAG)

The Scottish Office
NHS Executive
St Andrew's House
Regents Road
Edinburgh EH1 3DG

Clinical Governance Resource Centre for Dorset
Information and links to other sites.

http://www.bournemouth.ac.uk/schools/ihcs/clingov/index.htm

Clinical Evidence 99
A digest of best research findings on important clinical issues, updated 6 monthly. The first issue was due in book format in January 1999.

http://www.evidence.org

Clinical Guidelines: Using clinical guidelines to improve patient care within the NHS Executive
Describes how clinical guidelines should be developed, evaluated, implemented and monitored. Also lists organisations and other contacts and the guidelines developed to date. Produced by the Department of Health.

The Cochrane Collaboration
The Cochrane Collaboration is an organisation that rigorously examines and evaluates the evidence for particular clinical interventions. This is done through systematic reviews of the literature related to particular health-care issues, by a review group of experts, specially recruited to collaborate on a particular topic. This is the home page for this International Collaboration and provides access to information on its activities and the Handbook.

http://www.cochrane.org/cochrane/

The Cochrane Collaboration's Handbook
(See Cochrane Collaboration, above.) The main working document, in six parts to date. The first describes the background, aims and organisation of the Collaboration. The other five are aimed at those wishing to establish review groups or maintain randomised controlled trial and Cochrane Registers, so they are only for the more experienced clinician or academics.

http://hiru.mcmaster.ca/cochrane/cochrane/hbook.htm

Cochrane Effective Practice and Organisation of Care (EPOC) Group
Formerly known as Cochrane Collaboration on Effective Professional Practice (CCEPP). Information about the group, a newsletter, downloadable database of bibliographic references, plus links to health-related sites and information about discussion groups.

http://www.abdn.ac.uk/publichealth/hsru/epoc/index.htm

The Cochrane Library
An electronic publication of high-quality evidence to inform health-care decision-making. Published quarterly on CD-ROM, 3.5-inch diskettes and over the Internet. Includes: the Cochrane Database of Systematic Reviews (see above); Database of Abstracts of Reviews of Effectiveness (DARE – see above); the Cochrane Controlled Trials Register – bibliographic information on controlled trials; sources of information on the science of reviewing research and evidence-based health care. Subscription details and basic technical support available on the UK Cochrane Centre's website. A training package for the Cochrane Library is available, consisting of Powerpoint files and Word documents, including self-assessment exercises.

http://www.cochrane.org/cochrane/cdsr.htm

Abstracts of Cochrane Reviews
This site contains the titles of reviews and reviews in progress listed by the Collaborative Review Group. Access to the reviews themselves is password protected and only available by subscription.

http://hiru.mcmaster.ca/cochrane/cochrane/revabstr/abidx.htm

Core Library for Evidence-Based Practice
A list of books, reports and journals to act as a starting point. Intended for a library or clinical audit/effectiveness unit. See ScHARR.

Development and Evaluation Committee Reports
The Development and Evaluation Committee is funded by the Research and Development Directorate of the South and West region. The Committee examines health interventions at an early stage of their introduction, where the scientific evidence is new or

ambiguous and rates the weight of evidence for or against the intervention. The reports that it produces are intended to provide rapid, accurate and usable information to purchasers, clinicians, managers and researchers in the South and West in order to help them decide whether or in what circumstances the intervention should become standard practice. Reports are usually available in libraries, or from the South and West regional office.

http://www.hta.nhsweb.nhs.uk/rapidhta

Department of Health

As the statutory body responsible for health, the Department of Health (DoH) is the source of all policy decisions. The DoH maintains a website that lists organisations, publications, key documents and much else. It can take time to get to the subject you want, but it is comprehensive.

http://www.doh.gov.uk/dhome.htm

Eli Lilly National Clinical Audit Centre

Provides education, advice and information concerning clinical audit and effective practice for primary care.

Department of General Practice and Primary Healthcare
University of Leicester
Leicester General Hospital
Leicester LE5 4PW
Tel: 0116 258 4873

Evidence

Quarterly newsletter funded as a pilot scheme by the Welsh National Board for nursing, midwifery and health visiting educationalists.

School of Nursing and Midwifery Studies
Faculty of Health
University of Wales
Bangor

http://www.bangor.ac.uk/hs/evidence

Evidence-based Healthcare

The *Journal of Evidence-Based Health Care* aims to provide managers with the best available evidence about the financing, organisation and delivery of health care.

http://www.harcourt-international.com/journals/ebhc/

Evidence-based Healthcare – a resource pack

Contains reading and key references on the background and current thinking on evidence-based health care. Also has details of relevant groups and organisations. Designed to guide reading and aid contact with national organisations and academic bodies.

King's College School of Medicine and Dentistry
The Strand
London WC2R 2LS

http://drsdesk.sghms.ac.uk/Starnet/pack.htm

Evidence-based Medicine

The intention of this is to advise clinicians of advances in medicine, general and family practice, surgery, psychiatry, paediatrics, and obstetrics and gynaecology, by selecting from articles and reviews in the literature. These are then formally summarised in abstracts and commented on by clinical experts.

http://www.acponline.org/journals/ebm/ebmmenu.htm

Evidence-based Mental Health (EBMH)

Contains full text of the EBMH notebook, selected articles, archive of previous issues, journal purpose and policy, glossary of terms, letters, debates.

http://www.psychiatry.ox.ac.uk/cebmh/journal/

Evidence-based Nursing

This is published quarterly. It is an international journal summarising research evidence on a variety of nursing issues. Experts comment on each article, putting it into context, and point out the key research findings.

http://www.bmjpg.com/data/ebn.htm

Evidence-based Pathology

Developing at the University of Nottingham, this provides a gateway to EBM resources.

http://www.ccc.nottingham.ac.uk/~mpzjlowe/evpath.html

Evidence-based Purchasing

A bimonthly digest of evidence on effective care, intended to support the commissioning role of the health authorities. Consists of a selection of material received, commissioned, or found in journals by the South and West R&D Directorate.

Framework for Appropriate Care Throughout Sheffield (FACTS) Project

This is a city-wide project based in Sheffield, which aims to implement change in primary care. The first focus has been the use of aspirin for heart disease patients. A report, describing the methodology, lessons learned and broader implications for evidence-based change management, is available from the website.

Sheffield Centre for Health and Related Research
Regents Court
30 Regents Street
Sheffield S1 4DA
Tel: 0114 275 5658

http://www.shef.ac.uk/uni/projects/facts/

Health Evidence Bulletins, Wales

Information concerning best current evidence on health-care issues. Randomised controlled trials are included when available; otherwise evidence from high-quality observational and other studies. Topics so far include: maternal and early child health, oral health, respiratory diseases, mental health.

http://www.uwcm.ac.uk/uwcm/1b/pep/index.html

Healthcare Quality

Journal of the Association for Quality in Healthcare. Aims to improve the quality of healthcare through the dissemination of information about research, practical approaches and techniques. Also has a hotline, which is a free source of advice on health-care quality issues (0113 223 7296).

Health Technology Assessment (HTA) Database
Contains abstracts produced by INAHTA (International Network of Agencies for Health Technology Assessment) and other health-care technology agencies. Supported by the NHS Centre for Reviews and Dissemination at the University of York

http://nhscrd.york.ac.uk/

Health Technology Assessment Reports
Contains abstracts of completed reviews from the NHS Health Technology Assessment Programme located at Southampton University.

http://www.hta.nssweb.nhs.uk

Institute of Health Sciences, University of Oxford
A source of information on some useful publications, databases, web resources and organisations. Good links to other sites.

http://www.ihs.ox.ac.uk/

Institute of Psychiatry Library
De Crespigny Park
London SE5 8AF
Tel: 020 7919 3204
Fax: 020 7703 4515
Email: Spyllib@iop.bpmf.ac.uk

Journal of Advanced Nursing
Publishes papers related to all aspects of nursing – clinical practice, education, policy, management and research. This includes research reports, literature reviews, discussion. Published by Blackwell Scientific Press.

MIDIRS
The central point for databases, events, indexes, news and other information related to maternity care and childbirth.

http://www.midirs.org

The NHS Centre for Reviews and Dissemination (CRD)

A facility commissioned by the NHS Research and Development Division to produce and disseminate reviews on the effectiveness and cost-effectiveness of healthcare interventions. The aim is to identify, review and disseminate good quality health research to NHS decision and consumers. The reviews will cover: the effectiveness of care for particular conditions; the effectiveness of health technologies; evidence on efficient methods of organising and delivering particular types of healthcare. The CRD public databases are accessible over the Internet and via dial-up access. The first is a database of structured abstracts of good-quality systematic reviews *(DARE)* which, after rigorous scrutiny, comment on published reviews and summarise the conclusions and any implications for health practice. There is also an economic evaluations database *(NEED)*. The telnet address is nhscrd.york.ac.uk (the user ID and password are both crduser).

The Publications Office is:

NHS Centre for Reviews and Dissemination
University of York
York YO1 5DD

http://www.york.ac.uk/inst/crd/welcome.htm

National Institute for Clinical Excellence (NICE)

NICE was set up as a Special Health Authority in April 1999. It is accountable to the Secretaries of State for Health and for Wales and will promote clinical and cost-effectiveness, advise on best practice in the use of existing treatment options, including drugs, surgery, lifestyle, etc. NICE will also appraise new health treatments and advise the NHS on implementation. It will coordinate a number of other previous initiatives in disseminating information and responding to specific enquiries. NICE will work with other health organisations at a local level, such as NHS trusts, other service providers, health authorities, primary care groups (local health groups in Wales) and with patient representatives. NICE will have links with Royal Colleges, professional associations, academic units and health-care industries. It will also work with the Commission for Health Improvement.

NICE has incorporated the Effectiveness Bulletins – 'Effective Health Care' and 'Effectiveness Matters' – previously produced by the NHS Centre for Reviews and Dissemination (CRD), into its remit.

http://www.nice.org.uk/

National Centre for Clinical Audit (NCCA)
This has been linked into NICE. The NCCA is a resource for all healthcare professionals on all aspects of clinical audit. It maintains a database of audits undertaken, information on methodology, advice on undertaking audit and bringing about change and local and national contacts.

National Institute for Clinical Excellence
90 Long Acre
Covent Garden
London WC2 9RZ
Tel: 020 7849 3444

http://www.nice.org.uk

Nursing Standard Online
A weekly nursing journal published on the Internet.

Viking House
17–19 Peterborough Road
Harrow on the Hill
Middlesex HA1 2AX
Tel: 020 8423 1066
Fax 020 8423 3867

Email: nursingstandard@compuserve.com

Oxford and Anglia Mental Health Web (OXAMWEB)
Funded by the Directorate of Research and Development for the Anglia and Oxford Region, resources for Internet connection in libraries in the Region and for the development of OXAMWEB have been provided. Publications on OXAMWEB must meet clear criteria. Some material, marked by EB (evidence-based) logo, fulfils the more stringent criteria of evidence-based medicine.

http://cebmh.warne.ox.ac.uk/cebmh/nolmh

Promoting Action on Clinical Effectiveness (PACE)
This initiative is run from the King's Fund in London and aims to

achieve clinical change through 16 demonstration projects. A report is available from their site.

http://www.kingsfund.org.uk/

Promoting Clinical Effectiveness: A Framework for Action in and through the NHS (NHS Executive, 1996)
Sets out the basis for action for health authorities, trusts, healthcare professionals and patients in primary, secondary and community care.

Regional Offices home pages

All DoH Regional offices in England and Wales have undertaken to establish web pages. Those given below were the most up to date available after the alteration to Regional boundaries which took place in April 1999.

Eastern Regional Office
http://www.doh.gov.uk/ero/index.htm

London Regional Office
http://www.doh.gov.uk/london/home.htm

North West Region Office
http://www.doh.gov.uk/nwro/home.htm

North Yorkshire Region
http://www.doh.gov.uk/nyro/main/htm

South West Regional Office
http://www.doh.gov.uk/swro/swroh.htm

Trent Regional Office
http://nhstrent.users.netlink.co.uk/index.htm

West Midlands Regional Office
http://www.doh.gov.uk/wrmo/index.htm

Resources for Practising EBM
Many links to other sites. Specialises in paediatric critical care (aka intensive care) medicine. Has data-base, systematic reviews, critical

literature appraisal and bibliographies. Also includes the PedsCCM Evidence-based Journal Club.

http://pedsccm.wustl.edu/EBJ/EB_Resources.html

Royal College of Nursing and Midwifery Audit Information Service
Information service to support clinical effectiveness. Provides help in the location and appraisal of information, conducts literature searches, advises on standard setting and clinical audit, and has a contacts and projects database.

Royal College of Nursing
20 Cavendish Square
London WIM 0AF
Tel: 020 7629 7646

Royal College of Nursing Research and Development Co-ordinating Centre
Provides bibliography lists and other links.

School of Nursing, Midwifery and Health Visiting
University of Manchester
Gateway House
Piccadilly
Manchester M60 7LP

http://www.man.ac.uk/rcn/

Royal College of Nursing Library and Information Service
Contains 60 000 volumes and 500 videos, and receives 400 current periodicals on nursing and related subjects. Special collections include the Historical Collection and the Steinberg Collection of Nursing Research, comprising theses and dissertations on nursing subjects at Masters degree and PhD levels.

20 Cavendish Square
London W1M 0AB
Tel: 020 7647 3610 (Information Desk)
020 7647 3613 (Issue Desk)
Fax: 020 7647 3420

St George's Hospital Medical School Health Care Evaluation Unit

Department of Public Health Sciences
Cranmer Terrace
London SW17 0RE
Tel: 020 8725 2788

ScHARR-Lock's Guide to the Evidence

A guide to printed sources of evidence arranged by medical subject heading (MeSH), focusing on grey literature from UK academic and quasi-governmental sources.

http://www.shef.ac.uk/uni/academic/R-Z/scharr/ir/scebm.html

School of Health and Related Research (ScHARR), University of Sheffield

This is a health services research department within the University of Sheffield, which has expertise in literature searching; it provides critical appraisal training and systematic reviews has numerous links to other sites. The Information Resources Section produces a bibliography and resource guide *The ScHARR Guide to Evidence-based Practice*. A Microsoft Word Version 6 copy of this is available. Printed copies are available for £10.00 (inclusive of postage & packing) from:

ScHARR Information Resources
University of Sheffield
Regent Court
30 Regent Street
Sheffield, S1 4DA

http://www.shef.ac.uk/uni~scharr

UK Clearing House on Health Outcomes

The UK Clearing House on Health Outcomes is based in the Nuffield Institute for Health at the University of Leeds. It aims to develop approaches to outcomes assessment within routine healthcare practice and to promote the role of health outcomes in healthcare commissioning and provision. There are two databases available on the world-wide web: an outcomes database of structured abstracts and an outcomes activities database of outcomes-related projects. This enables networking of people working in similar areas or using similar measures.

Nuffield Institute for Health
71–75 Clarendon Road
Leeds LS2 9PL
Tel: 0113 233 3940

http://www.leeds.ac.uk/nuffield/infoservices/UKCH/home.html

Index